Defeat
Osteoporosis

Dr Sushil Sharma

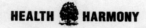

HEALTH HARMONY

An imprint of

B. Jain Publishers (P) Ltd.

An ISO 9001 : 2000 Certified Company

USA — Europe — India

DEFEAT OSTEOPOROSIS

First Edition: 2010
1st Impression: 2010

All rights reserved. No part of this book may be reproduced, stored in a retrieval system or transmitted, in any form or by any means, mechanical, photocopying, recording or otherwise, without any prior written permission of the publisher.

© with the author

Published by Kuldeep Jain for
HEALTH 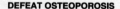 HARMONY
An imprint of
B. JAIN PUBLISHERS (P) LTD.
An ISO 9001 : 2000 Certified Company
1921/10, Chuna Mandi, Paharganj, New Delhi 110 055 (INDIA)
Tel.: +91-11-4567 1000 • *Fax:* +91-11-4567 1010
Email: info@bjain.com • *Website:* **www.bjainbooks.com**

Printed in India

ISBN: 978-81-319-0663-7

DEDICATION

Dedicated to my father Late Shri J.P. Sharma

FOREWORD

The 'Defeat Osteoporosis' book for disseminating knowledge about osteoporosis to general masses is a very positive and people friendly step and I congratulate the Arthritis Foundation of India and Dr Sushil Sharma, Chairman, AFI for it.

Osteoporosis is an under-recognised disease and symptoms appear usually after the damage has been done. This is precisely the reason why people need to be sensitised about various aspects of the disease.

India is a huge country with multiple sub-cultures, various castes, religions, languages and therefore AFI's work is not easy at all. But its inclusive and comprehensive approach has already started showing results. I am extremely confident that this easy-to-understand book will go a long way in realisation of IOF's and AFI's goal of an osteoporosis-free India. I recommend it as a compulsory reading for all those who are interested in strong bones.

Prof. John A. Kanis
International Osteoporosis Foundation President
Director, WHO Collaborating Centre

PREFACE

The saying 'Prevention is better than cure' holds good in all times. But for prevention we need knowledge about the disease. Osteoporosis is a silent disease which creeps into our bones like a thief and steals all the strength leading to fractures. Millions of people are already suffering from this disease in India and worldwide; and millions are in the queue. WHO realised the gigantic problem and declared 2000 to 2010 as bone and joint decade.

The AFI conducted a survey in 2006-07 in The National Capital Territory of Delhi to know the level of awareness about osteoporosis among people. The results were startling and truly an eye opener. Less than 10 percent of people knew about osteoporosis as a disease entity and a major cause of fractures. This convinced us at AFI about the need for a large scale awareness activity. Thus, comes the raison d'être for a book on osteoporosis, which is meant to inform the general reader. The main objective is to tell everybody that 'you are the master of your bones so take care, take control'.

The AFI slogan 'Bone Health is a Right, Realise It' is very pertinent. This disease is preventable, treatable and controllable to a large extent and therefore people should refuse to suffer. Begin today starting from your own bones then move on to your family. God bless you all on this fascinating journey.

Yours' sincerely
Dr Sushil Sharma
Chairman, AFI

ACKNOWLEDGEMENT

I sincerely feel indebted to thousands of fracture and osteoporosis patients whose pain and agony has sensitised and motivated me for this small service towards the 'common man'.

Thanks to International Osteoporosis Foundation family and especially Prof. Cyrus Cooper, Chairman Scientific Committee, IOF for their encouragement. I am grateful to Prof. P.K. Dave, former Director AIIMS and I express my gratitude to AFI's scientific committee Prof. Shishir Rastogi, Dr Anil Arora, Dr Prateek Gupta and Dr Atul Kakkar for their positive suggestions and careful reviews. Thanks for the helpful activism about bone health to Mr Harsh Sharma, Mr Kailash Jain and Mr Dharam R. Pawar.

Tons of thanks to Dr Seema, Paediatrician, Trustee AFI and my wife for the valuable solicited inputs, my children Pakhi and Sarthak, who sanctioned me enough time to finish the job in the stipulated period. Thanks to my mother Mrs. Maya Devi for pushing me towards social work.

Thanks to Richa, Personnel Manager AFI for the office support and nutritionist Shikha Bhargava and Deepika Kohli in finalising dietary schedules. Last but not the least thanks to Dr Akshay Saxena for helping me in finalising the book.

Dr Sushil Sharma
Sr. Orthopaedic Surgeon and Chairman
Arthritis Foundation of India Trust

WHAT DRIVES ME TO WRITE THIS BOOK

AFI survey about arthritis and osteoporosis awareness

A survey was conducted by AFI on a sample size of 1000 people in the month of April, May and June, 2007 as part of epidemiological community based research.

Survey conclusions

		Result
Q1. How many people know that Osteoporosis and Arthritis are different disease entities?		**36.5%**
i.	Men above 40	38.2%
ii.	Men below 40	41.2%
iii.	Women above 40	40.1%
iv.	Women below 40	23.4%
Q2. How many people know that Arthritis is of different types?		**36.2%**
i.	Men above 40	35.8%
ii.	Men below 40	33.7%
iii.	Women above 40	58.1%
iv.	Women below 40	28.2%
Q3. How many people know that Arthritis is a disease of all age groups?		**7.7%**
i.	Men above 40	6.4%
ii.	Men below 40	3.9%
iii.	Women above 40	7.4%
iv.	Women below 40	4.7%

Q4. How many people know that Osteoporosis is treatable? **46.4%**

  i. Men above 40 — 41.6%
  ii. Men below 40 — 55.5%
  iii. Women above 40 — 48.3%
  iv. Women below 40 — 35.4%

Q5. How many people know that Arthritis can be treated successfully? **34.4%**

  i. Men above 40 — 32.4%
  ii. Men below 40 — 40.1%
  iii. Women above 40 — 41.8%
  iv. Women below 40 — 22.4%

Q6. How many people know that in Arthritis operation is helpful? **33.1%**

  i. Men above 40 — 32.4%
  ii. Men below 40 — 36.9%
  iii. Women above 40 — 38.5%
  iv. Women below 40 — 23.9%

Q7. How many people know that majority of fractures are basically complications of Osteoporosis? **10.05%**

  i. Men above 40 — 11.9%
  ii. Men below 40 — 9.8%
  iii. Women above 40 — 13.9%
  iv. Women below 40 — 7.6%

Q8. How many people know that Osteoporosis is treatable with medicines alone and no surgery is required? **39.0%**

  i. Men above 40 — 33.1%
  ii. Men below 40 — 50.7%
  iii. Women above 40 — 36.0%
  iv. Women below 40 — 27.7%

PUBLISHER'S NOTE

With the increasing modernisation and changing lifestyle, people are becoming more vulnerable to diseases. With lack of awareness and non-reactive attitude towards diseases and disorders, it becomes very essential to spread the information to help the masses lead a longer and healthy life.

Osteoporosis is a very common ailment affecting both males and females. People usually neglect their initial symptoms and tend to suffer later on. Prevention is better than cure, the old adage points out rightly. With active lifestyle and proper balanced diet, osteoporosis can be avoided and the person can lead a healthier life.

This book 'Defeat Osteoporosis' is an attempt by the author to share his knowledge and also clinical experience in order to make the common man conscious of the disease and its related information ranging from symptomatology to diagnosis, treatment and also prevention.

It gives me immense pleasure to present this book in an attempt to help people deal with osteoporosis but the emphasis is to prevent the disease at first place.

Kuldeep Jain
C.E.O., B. Jain Publishers (P) Ltd.

CONTENTS

Foreword .... *iii*
Preface .... *v*
Acknowledgement .... *vii*
What Drives me to Write this Book .... *ix*
Publisher's Note .... *xiii*

1. Introduction 1
2. The Architecture of The Bones 11
3. Osteoporosis 17
4. Falls and Fractures 33
5. Exercise and Bones 39
6. Nutrition 47
7. Life style 55
8. The Treatment of Osteoporosis 59
9. Bone Health in School Children 73
10. The Value of Milk 85
11. Bone Health at Work Place 91
12. OTC Drugs 93
13. Case History of Patients 97
14. Physiotherapy Gadgets 105
15. Recipes 113
16. Alternative Therapies 155
    • Homeopathy

- Herbal remedies
- Ayurveda
- Chinese herbs
- Yoga
- Acupuncture
- Home remedies

Appendix – I to V 165

DISCLAIMER

Alternative therapy section of the book and the related information has been compiled for the readers' benefit by the editors of B.Jain Publishers.

Chapter 1
Introduction

Brief Historical Background

The Egyptian mummies and the ancient cadaveric observations have revealed osteoporosis and thinning of bones. Historical commentators say that many legendary characters in history were bedridden in their later years following hip fractures. So, the disease is as old as human beings but the knowledge about the ailment is new.

Age Factor - East v/s West

Myth or a fact

The average age at death in India is 64 while the average longevity in Europe is 79 in men, 84 in women and that in USA is 78. Although the average age in West is higher, still osteoporosis is more prevalent in India, reason being the disease strikes here at a much younger age, that is, 40's and 50's. One can imagine the disease load if the average age becomes at par with the west. With improvement in general healthcare longevity in India is also increasing which will result in exponential increase in osteoporotic patients.

Despite the looming threat osteoporosis has become, Government efforts to tackle the menace has been far from encouraging. If India wants to be a super-power, its people must be in perfect health. The Arthritis Foundation of India wants India and the world free from osteoporosis. In this process, it issues a call for proactive action from both the Government as well as the people.

Definition of Osteoporosis by WHO

'A systemic skeletal disorder characterised by a low bone mass and microarchitectural deterioration of bone tissue, with a subsequent increase in bone fragility and susceptibility to fracture'.

The International Osteoporosis Foundation (IOF)

The International Osteoporosis Foundation (IOF), registered as a not-for-profit, non-governmental foundation in Switzerland, functions as a global alliance of patients, medical and research societies, scientists, health care professionals and international companies concerned about bone health. IOF headquarters are in Nyon, Switzerland, with a second secretariat located in Lyon, France.

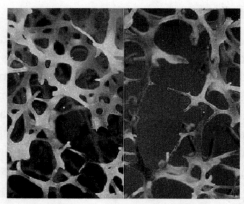

Fig. 1.1(a) Normal Bone   Fig. 1.1(b) Osteoporotic Bone

The Foundation was established in 1998, when the European Foundation for Osteoporosis (EFFO), founded in 1987, joined with the International Federation of Societies on Skeletal Diseases (IFSSD, established 1995).

The new IOF one-minute osteoporosis risk test

This is the self-help test by which any person can know for him or herself the level of risk to bones. There are nineteen easy questions to help you understand the status of your bone health.

What you cannot change

Family History

i. Have either of your parents been diagnosed with osteoporosis or broken a bone after a minor fall (a fall from standing height or less)?

   Yes / No

ii. Did either of your parents have a 'dowager's hump'?

   Yes / No

   Personal clinical factors

   These are fixed risk factors that one is born with or cannot alter but, that is not to say that they should be ignored. It is important to be aware of fixed risks so that steps can be taken to reduce loss of bone mineral.

iii. Are you 40 years old or older?

   Yes / No

iv. Have you ever broken a bone after a minor fall, as an adult?

   Yes / No

v. Do you fall frequently (more than once in the last year) or do you have a fear of falling because you are frail?

   Yes / No

vi. After the age of 40, have you lost more than 3 cm in height (just over 1 inch)?
Yes / No

vii. Are you underweight (is your Body Mass Index less than 19 kg/m^2)?
Yes / No

How to calculate your Body Mass Index (BMI)

Body mass index (BMI) is a measure based on height and weight that applies to both adult men and women.

BMI = Weight (kilogram)/ Height (metre^2)

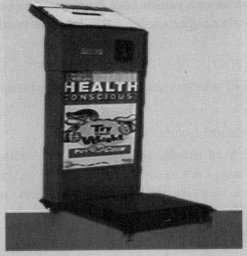

Fig. 1.2 BMI Machine

BMI Categories

Underweight = below 18.5

Normal weight = 18.5 – 24.9

Overweight = 25 – 29.9

Obesity = 30 or greater

Imperial BMI Formula

The imperial BMI formula accepts weight measurements in pounds and height measurements in either inches or feet.

1 foot = 12 inches

Inches^2 = inches x inches

Metric BMI Formula

The metric BMI formula accepts weight measurements in kilograms and height measurements in either centimetre or metres.

1 meter = 100 cm.

Meters^2 = meters x meters

viii. Have you ever taken corticosteroid tablets (cortisone, prednisolone, etc.) for more than 3 consecutive months (corticosteroids are often prescribed for conditions like asthma, rheumatoid arthritis, and some inflammatory diseases)?

Yes / No

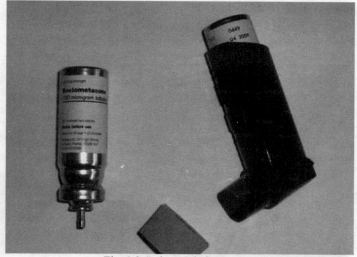

Fig. 1.3 Asthma Inhaler

ix. Have you ever been diagnosed with rheumatoid arthritis?
Yes / No

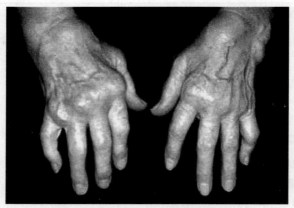

Fig. 1.4 Rheumatoid arthritis

x. Have you been diagnosed with an over-reactive thyroid or over-reactive parathyroid gland?

Yes / No

For women

For women over 45

xi. Did your menopause occur before the age of 45?

Yes / No

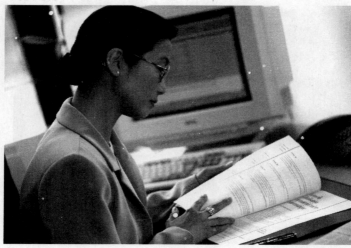

For working women aged 45 years

xii. Have your periods ever stopped for twelve consecutive months or more (other than because of pregnancy, menopause or hysterectomy)?

Yes / No

xiii. Were your ovaries removed before the age of fifty, without you taking Hormone Replacement Therapy?

Yes / No

For men

xiv. Have you ever suffered from impotency, lack of libido or other symptoms related to low testosterone levels?

Yes / No

What you can change

Lifestyle factors or modifiable risk factors which primarily arise because of diet or lifestyle choices.

xv. Do you regularly drink alcohol in excess of safe drinking limits (more than 2 units a day – 1 unit is 30 ml.)?

Yes / No

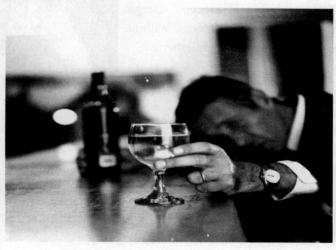

xvi. Do you currently, or have you ever, smoked cigarettes?

Yes / No

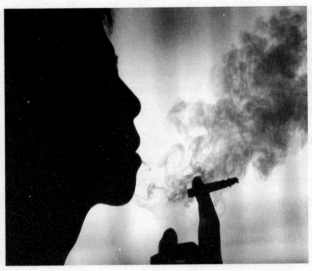

xvii. Is your daily level of physical activity less than thirty minutes (housework, gardening, walking, running etc.)?

Yes / No

xviii. Do you avoid or are you allergic to milk or dairy products, without taking any calcium supplements?

Yes / No

xix. Do you spend less than ten minutes per day outdoors (with part of your body exposed to sunlight), without taking vitamin D supplements?

Yes / No

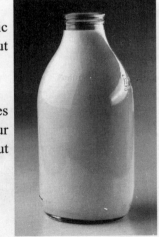

Understanding your answers

If you answered 'yes' to any of these questions it does not mean that you have osteoporosis. Positive answers simply mean that you have clinically-proven risk factors which may lead to osteoporosis and fractures.

Please show this risk test to your physician or health care professional who may encourage you to have a Bone Mineral Density test (BMD) and who will advise on what treatment, if any, is recommended.

If you have no or few risk factors you should nevertheless discuss your bone health with your physician and monitor your risks in the future. You should also discuss osteoporosis with your family and friends and encourage them to take this test.

Chapter 2
The Architecture of the Bones

The skeleton consists of 206 bones and constitutes 15 percent of total body weight. The functions of bones are to support, locomotion, protection of body parts, store house of minerals (90 percent of calcium, 85 percent of phosphorus, 50 percent of magnesium) and it also acts as store house of bone matrix proteins such as collagens and bone morphogenic proteins etc. Skeleton can be divided into two components:

i. **Axial skeleton**–refers to back and hip joint area and this area is primarily spongy having high turn over.
ii. **Appendicular skeleton**–refers to long bones of leg and arm primarily hard with low turn over.

The bone has two main functions to perform: weight bearing and flexibility. The specific structural macroscopic and microscopic organisation is responsible for it by virtue of its configuration, bone size, proportion of compact (cortical) to cancellous bone, lamellar organisation of bony tissue, degree of mineralisation of bony tissue and cable like organization of collagen molecules and their cross linking.

Protein of bone comprises of special mixture that is, matrix (material laid down by bone forming cells) made up of layers of collagen molecules between which crystalline calcium and phosphorus are deposited. Gradually the bone mineralises and mineral density increases as it gets older.

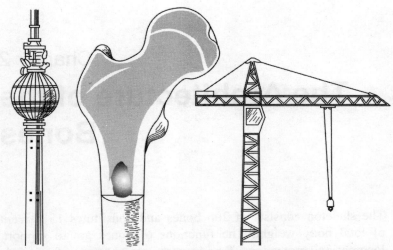

Fig. 2.1 Architectural organisation of femoral head, neck, and shaft, combining the two principles of construction for maximal weight bearing tubular structure illustrated by the television tower and trabecular structure by the crane
(Source- Bartl and Frisch osteoporosis)

New matrix begins to mineralise in 5–10 days (primary mineralisation). After remodeling gradual maturation of mineral components takes place (secondary mineralisation). Collagen is responsible for the elasticity and flexibility of bone while minerals provide strength and rigidity. Degree of mineralisation depends on rate of remodeling.

Radiologically as we see on x-ray two main supporting structures can be identified:

i. Compact, cortical bone
ii. Spongy, cancellous, trabecular bone

Cortical bone is outer layer of long bone. It is very dense and has slow metabolic rate so it is slow to heal if it gets fractured, seen in cases of long bones like femur and humerus. While in cancellous bone randomly distributed trabeculae along the line of stress and weight bearing (trajection lines) can be seen, producing sponge like structures, for example, in axial skeleton (cranium, vertebral column, thorax and pelvis).

The Architecture of the Bones

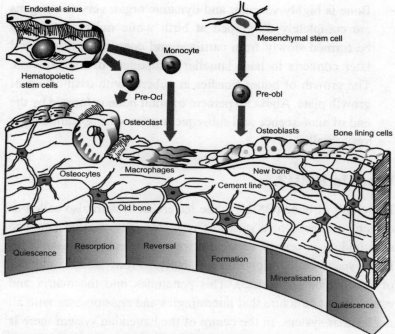

Fig. 2.2 Steps of bone remodelling in adult trabecular bone.
(The total quantity of bone decreases if more bone is resorbed over years than is produced. It has been estimated that osteoporosis develops, when for every 30 units of bone resorbed only 29 are produced.)
(Source- Bartl and Frisch osteoporosis)

The cortical bone has three surfaces and each has different anatomic features. The inner most is called endosteal envelop which faces the marrow cavity and has high turn over. Intracortical envelop forms the middle layer consisting the haversian system. The periosteal envelop forms the outer most layer to which ligaments, tendon and muscles are attached.

- Approximately 80 percent bone is cortical and only 20 percent is trabecular
- About 25 percent of cancellous bone is remodeled annually while only 2.5 percent of cortical bone goes through the process

- Bone is highly vascular and dynamic organ very few organs are completely developed at birth while most continue to be formed slowly from cartilage and connective tissues and later converts to hard lamellar component of the skeleton. The growth of bones finishes at puberty with ossification of growth plate. About 90 percent of adult bone is formed by the end of adolescence and subsequent gains during adulthood is very small.

What is BMU?

Basic unit of bone (BMU) is the haversian system also called as osteon. It consist of a series of concentrically parallel lamellae surrounding a central canal. Between the lamellae, osteocytes lie in space called Howship's Lacunae. From lacunae number of canaliculae are formed. This penetrates into the matrix and establishes a structure that intermingles and anastomoses with all the lacunar system. In the centre of the haversian system there is a central canal varying between 2-8 mm in length and filled with interlacing tissue, osteoblasts and osteocytes.

The bone is normally surrounded by periosteum, which consists of two layers, an outer layer of elastic tissue and an inner layer called cambium. Elastic tissue is the only layer of periosteum on intra articular surface of neck of femur. Periosteum also provides mechanism by which muscles are attached to bone and normally at these sites there is increased vascularity of bone itself.

Dynamic Bone Parameters
- 3-4 million BMU initiated per year
- 1 million BMU operating at any given moment
- BMU about 1-2 mm long and 0.2-0.4mm wide
- Life span of BMU about 6-9 months

The Architecture of the Bones

- Speed of BMU about 25µm/day
- Lifespan of active osteoblast about 3 months
- Lifespan of active osteoclast about 2weeks
- Interval between successive remodeling events at same site about 2-5 years
- Rate of turn over of whole skeleton about 10% per year
- BMU = Basic Multicellular Unit in Bone

During childhood there is a continuous process of remodeling which maintains the skeleton and adapts bone to changing external environments. As the bone ages it loses its strength and elasticity, it is due to change in bone matrix. Bone undergoes constant removal and formation.

Remodeling consists of mobilisation of calcium in the frame work, replacement of old osseous tissue, skeletal adaptation to different loads, weight bearing and stress and repair of damaged bone both microscopic and macroscopic.

Wolff's Law–Putting stress on the bones causes them to form more bone and lack of stress on bone causes bone loss.

The bone cells constitute a specialised osseous cell system responsible for repair and adaptation of bone. The various exercise regimes are basically designed considering this law.

Types of cells

i. **Osteoclasts (bone breaker or bone carvers)**–Can reabsorb old bone in a short period of time. These multi nucleated giant cells are derived from monocytes of bone marrow. The cell membrane of these cells consists of numerous folds–the ruffled border faces the surface of bone. Osteoclasts release proteolytic and other enzymes into the ruffled folds and these dissolve bone matrix, rest is phagocytosed and metabolised into cytoplasm. Recruitment of osteoclasts is done by various hormones as paratharmone, oestrogen, leptin, thyroid hormone as well as cytokinins.

ii. **Osteoblast (bone builders)**—Derived from mesenchyme in the bone marrow they produce new bone over several weeks time. Their main function is to synthesise bone matrix, especially collagen Type-1 and also bone morphogenic proteins.

iii. **Osteocytes (bone maintainers)**—These are most numerous in all bone cells and they develop from osteoblasts. Approximately every tenth osteoblast becomes an osteocyte. It has receptor for PTH and sex hormone. Osteocytes occupy space in the bone called lacunae and are connected to each other and to the surface of the bone by thin channels called canaliculi within which long cytoplasmic processes join osteocytes to each other thus, forming the circulatory system. They also possess functional gap junctions enabling them to communicate with one another. So they are able to pass load induced signals to preosteoblasts which then differentiate and secrete osteoid. They play an important role in transport of organic and inorganic material in the bone.

Chapter 3
Osteoporosis

The IOF Definition
'Osteoporosis is a disease in which the density and quality of bone are reduced, leading to weakness of the skeleton and increased risk of fracture, particularly of the spine, wrist, hip, pelvis and upper arm. Osteoporosis and fractures are an important cause of mortality and morbidity'.

The WHO Definition
Osteoporosis is defined as a *'disease characterised by low bone mass and micro-architectural deterioration of bone tissue, leading to enhanced bone fragility and a consequent increase in fracture risk. It is characterised by generalised reduction in bone mass due to sub-normal osteoid production, excessive rate of deossification and sub-normal osteoid mineralisation'.* It has also been defined as a *'bone mineral density that is below the age adjusted reference range or more than one standard deviation below the mean for a particular age'.*

On the basis of the modified classification by Nordin (1964), which on account of findings by the World Health Organisation (WHO) on causes of generalised and secondary osteoporosis, osteoporosis can be generalised or localised.

Generalised Osteoporosis

Primary

On the basis of patterns of bone loss and fracture, Riggs and Melton (1988) identified two types of primary osteoporosis:

i. **Type I** primary osteoporosis is post menopausal or osteoclast mediated

ii. **Type II** primary osteoporosis is senile or osteoblast mediated

Type I primary osteoporosis is characterised by a rapid bone loss seen in recent post menopausal women. The turnover of trabecular bone is accelerated. Therefore, distal radial and vertebral fractures are common.

Type II osteoporosis is characterised by age related bone loss, calcium deficiency and / or hyperparathyroidism. Variations have been observed in the ratio of incidence among men and women in different parts of the world. Fractures of the proximal femur, especially fracture of the neck of femur and intertrochanteric fractures are more common in this type of osteoporosis.

Secondary

The causes of generalised secondary osteoporosis in adults can be classified as hormonal, nutritional, drugs related to mineral metabolism, inherited metabolic disorders and other causes.

i. Hormonal

- Hypogonadism
- Hyperadrenocorticism
- Thyrotoxicosis
- Hyperprolactinaemia
- Adult hypophosphatasia
- Diabetes mellitus

Let us discuss the common causes –

Diabetes and osteoporosis

Diabetes is of two types—Type I starts at young age, mostly insulin injections are required, kidney damage (ketoacidosis) is more common. Insulin generating beta cells are scarce.

Early onset of diabetes in patients of Type I is usually associated with low bone mass. This may appear to be due to impaired osteoblastic nutrition and function. It can also be confirmed by decreased blood marker such as osteo calcin.

In contrast Type II diabetes does not have low bone mass, bone turn over may be suppressed in patients with poor sugar control. It is noted that higher fracture risk is present in Type II diabetes patients despite normal bone mass because of falls. The reason being neuropathy resulting in lack of sensation in feet, impaired vision, lack of coordination, poor muscle control and obesity.

Type II diabetes is ailment of elderly age group, usually above forty, the beta cells are not so scarce, most of the patients can be handled with oral hypoglycaemic agents and the chances of kidney damage(ketoacidocis) are less.

Thyrotoxicosis and osteoporosis

Thyroid disease falls into two major functional categories–

a. Conditions that produce too little thyroid hormone (hypothyroidism)
b. Conditions that produce too much thyroid hormone (hyperthyroidism)

In general, excessive replacement of thyroid hormone in medications can also result in signs and symptoms of hyperthyroidism. One of the problems that occurs when the thyroid is too active, or when too much thyroid hormone medication is given, is bone loss from osteoporosis.

Osteoporosis is the thinning of bone mass (decrease in bone density), which leads to fragile bones that can break more easily.

There are a number of contributing factors for osteoporosis, including heredity, the amount of peak bone mass acquired during youth and factors that contribute to an increased breakdown of bone and/or a decrease in the formation of new bone. Hyperthyroidism is associated with an increased excretion of calcium and phosphorus in the urine and stool, which results in a loss of bone mineral. This loss is documented by the measurement of bone density (densitometry) and leads to an increased risk of broken bones (fractures). If the hyperthyroidism is treated early, bone loss can be minimised. In the same manner, excessive amounts of thyroid hormone replacement medication can also result in bone loss.

In addition to osteoporosis, hyperthyroidism can cause blood calcium levels to rise (hypercalcaemia) by as much as 25 percent. Occasionally, this may be severe enough to cause a stomach upset, excessive urination and impaired kidney function.

What do you need to know?

If you are on thyroid replacement medication, it is important to have your thyroid blood levels checked regularly to ensure that the appropriate amount of medication is taken. If you have a history of hyperthyroidism and are concerned that you may have osteoporosis, discuss the role of a bone density scan with your doctor. The level of calcium in the blood can easily be determined through a routine blood test.

If you have osteoporosis, there are many medications in the market that help to prevent further bone loss and can actually help to rebuild bone mass. Your doctor can guide you through the choices available.

ii. Nutritional

- Gastric surgery (total gastrectomy)
- Malabsorption syndrome/ malnutrition
- Calcium deficiency
- Alcoholism (discussed later)
- Chronic liver disease
- Scurvy (Vitamin C deficiency)
- Vitamin D deficiency

iii. Drugs

- Chronic heparin administration
- Vitamin D toxicity
- Anticonvulsants

Epilepsy and Osteoporosis

We would like to draw your attention to a recent publication which establishes a link between some anti-epileptic drugs and decreased bone mineral density. The anti-epileptic drugs which may pose a risk are: carbamazepine, phenytoin, primidone, phenobarbital and sodium valproate. Long term use of these drugs may lead to a higher risk of decreased bone mineral density which on the other hand may lead to osteopenia, osteoporosis and increased fractures for 'at risk' patients. Those classified as 'at risk' include people who have been inactive for long periods or have a lack of calcium in their diet. It is recommended that 'at risk' patients who are taking drugs for a long term consider taking Vitamin D supplements. At the moment there is not enough data to support a link between decreased bone mineral density and other antiepileptic drugs. The necessary measures can be taken for osteoporosis without disturbing the anti epilepsy treatment schedule.

iv. Inherited metabolic disorders

- Inherited disorder of collagen metabolism
- Ehler-Danlo's syndrome

- Osteogenesis imperfecta
- Homocystinuria due to cystathionine deficiency
- Marfan's syndrome

v. Other causes
- Porphyrinuria
- Thalassemia
- Generalised rheumatoid arthritis
- Anorexia nervosa (intake is very less)
- Myeloma and some cancers
- Space flight (due to weightlessness)
- Pregnancy
- Systemic mastocytosis

Localised Secondary Osteoporosis

The factors which give rise to localised secondary osteoporosis can be identified as:

- A prolonged immobilisation of a limb, for example in a plaster cast or high dorsal paraplegia/ low cervical quadriplegia. This form of osteoporosis is known as disuse osteoporosis.
- Monoarticular rheumatoid arthritis
- Sudeck's osteodystrophy

The clinical recognition of osteoporosis has changed over the last two decades. Definitions of the WHO now recognise moderate and marked reductions in bone density with the terms osteopenia and osteoporosis respectively.

Osteopenia is defined as a bone density between 1 and 2.5 standard deviations below the mean value in young adults. Osteoporosis has a bone density more than 2.5 standard deviations below the normal mean.

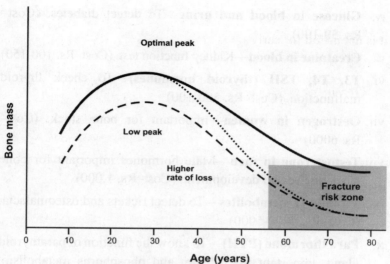

Fig. 3.1 Relation of loss of Bone Mass with age (years)

Investigations Relevant in Osteoporosis

The parameters of blood and urine test are within normal limits in genetically predisposed osteoporosis. Basically laboratory tests are for identification of secondary osteoporosis, that is, one which is due to an acquired cause.

List of laboratory tests

i. **CBC**—It's an indicator for poor food absorption in intestines and bone cancer. (Cost–Rs. 300)

ii. **Calcium and Phosphate level in blood**—Can give information about deficiency in the bone called osteomalacia, intestinal diseases related with food absorption, hyperparathyroidism. (Cost–Rs. 200-300)

iii. **Alkaline Phosphatase level in blood**—To diagnose rickets and osteomalacia. (Cost–Rs. 100)

iv. **Glucose in blood and urine**—To detect diabetes. (Cost–Rs. 50-100)
v. **Creatnine in blood**—Kidney function test. (Cost–Rs. 100-150)
vi. **T3, T4, TSH (thyroid hormones)**—To check thyroid malfunction. (Cost–Rs. 500-100)
vii. **Oestrogen in women**—Important for bone stock. (Cost–Rs. 6000)
viii. **Testosterone in men**—Male hormones important for bone stock and sexual development. (Cost–Rs. 1,000)
ix. **Vitamin D metabolites**—To detect rickets and osteomalacia. (Cost–Rs. 4000-5000)
x. **Para thormone (PTH)**—To know the function of parathyroid gland, important for calcium and phosphorus metabolism. (Cost–Rs. 1000-1200)
xi. **Protein electrophoresis**—To check certain bone cancers like multiple myeloma. (Cost–Rs. 500)
xii. Deoxypyridinoline (DPD)—One of the test to know osteoporosis. (Cost–Rs. 2900)
xiii. **Bone Markers**
- They are enzymes (chemicals) involved in bone formation or by-porducts (proteins) from bone resorption. They are not for diagnosis of Osteoporosis. They are checked in blood and urine.
- Bone specific Alkaline phosphatase (ALP) and Osteocalcin are parameters of bone formation
- Deoxypyridinoline and Cross linked telopeptides of type 1 collagen are two frequently checked
- Bone markers give early idea about improved bone density than DEXA scan say in 3-6 months (approximate Cost Rs. 5000)

xiv. **X-Rays**—X-rays can show the bone loss when the density of the bone is reduced by 30-40 percent, it is not useful for early detection and quantification of osteoporosis. Nevertheless, in case of spine osteoporosis which leads to compression (reduction in the height) of vertebrae can be detected by X-rays. So is the case with other fractures. It is less expensive and is a readily available tool in the hands of physicians. (Cost–Rs. 80-150 / Film; Digital X-Ray Rs. 250-350 / Film.)

xv. **CT Scan**—CT scan can be a good gadget for visualization of spongy bone but is not good for detecting the bone density. (Cost approximately Rs. 2,000.)

xvi. **MRI**—MRI is excellent for detecting various conditions related to bone marrow and adjoining nerves and tissues but not for bone density. (Cost–Rs. 5,000 to 6,000).

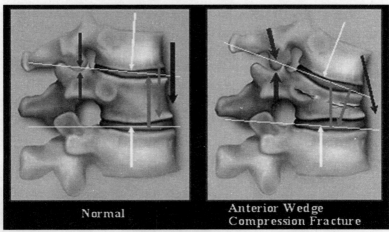

Fig. 3.2 Loss of Vertebral height in Osteoporosis

xvii. **BMD**—Bone mineral densitometry measurements can be done by Dexa scan, Ultrasound based scans (BMD machines) but Dexa scan is considered to be gold standard. BMD can detect osteoporosis irrespective of the cause.

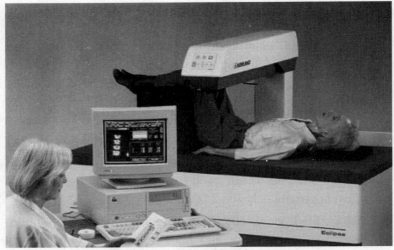

Fig. 3.3 Bone Mineral Densitometry

Bone Mineral Density estimation is considered best for prediction of fracture risk and therefore the treatment measures are mainly directed towards increasing the bone mineral density. A 10 percent decrease in bone density doubles the fracture risk for vertebral body and triples for the hip joint. In cases where a patient has sustained a fracture, a BMD test will not only confirm the diagnosis of osteoporosis but also the improvement in bone density can be checked again after six months to watch for reduction of second fracture risk.

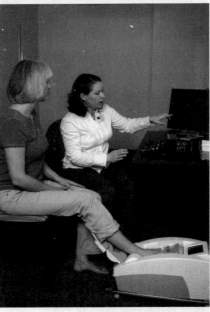

Fig. 3.4 Heel Based Unit

Outcome of treatment is to have stronger bones, but to achieve a normal BMD value for an osteoporotic patient may not be possible. The cost of Dexa scan (BMD Test) in the market for hip and spine is approximately Rs. 2,500-3,000. The ultra-sound based machines are also good diagnostic tools mainly used for screening camps, therefore, many a times manual errors are reported.

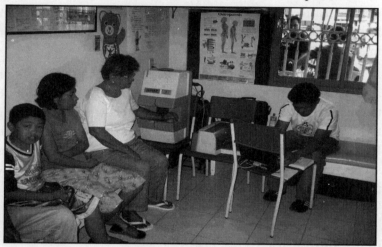

Fig. 3.5 Wrist Based Unit

WHO classification of reduction in bone density

Bone Mineral Density measured by BMD machine as follows:

T Score	Inference
> -1	Normal
(-1) – (-2.5)	Osteopenia (Less weak bone)
< (-2.5)	Osteoporosis (Very weak bone)

T Score is standard bone density of young adult. There is one Z – score, which is an age related scale but for all practical purposes T Score is taken as guide.

Off The Beat – Osteoporosis

Reflex Sympathetic Dystrophy (RSD)

It is an unusual medical condition, may occur in limbs, post trauma, where apparently there is a disturbance to vegetative nervous system in affected areas, most commonly in knee, ankle, forearm, hand and foot injury. The severity of injury has no bearing on intensity of RSD.

At times even doctors are unable to comprehend the condition as it is not easily explained, owing to exaggerated response to trauma. Patient definitely is lost and wonders what is happening to him or her. Apparently sometimes a small looking injury or fracture results in swelling and pain for months and years. At times skepticism drives them to various consultants and unnecessarily they keep on spending money.

The three phases of RSD are-

i. Inflammatory

- Phase 0-3 months
- Skin bluish, tense, swollen, restricted movements of joints
- X-ray yields no extra finding

ii. Dystrophic stage

- 3-6 months
- Swelling reduces but trophic (dry, cracked) skin appears

iii. Atrophic stage

- 6-12 months
- Atrophy of skin, muscle and bone

- X-ray picture shows washed out appearance of bone, that is, severe osteoporosis

Recovery is spontaneous and stages may not follow the same path. Besides oral Calcium and Vitamin D along with Bisphosphonate is prescribed. The intravenous injections of Bisphosphonates are of great help.

Gorham – Stout Syndrome

Ultimate severe Osteoporosis vanishing bones has angiogenic (blood vessels) related etiology. Not many cases of this type are reported in general, fortunately.

Steroids: The Biggest Enemy of Bones

The glucocorticoid therapy in form of tablets, injections and aerosol puffs (inhalers) for sniffing, if taken all together for longer periods – generally more than 6 months, may lead to osteoporosis and depletion of bone stock. They are generally taken by body builders and patients of bronchial asthma, lung diseases, skin ailments, auto immune diseases like rheumatoid arthritis, arthopathies, intestinal absorption disease like Crohn's disease, ulcerative colitis, multiple myeloma (Cancer) and other blood cancer like lymphoma. The kidney, liver organ transplant patients also need to be watchful. Mostly steroids intake leads to bone loss up to 20% in a year and a fallout results into a fracture at any area like hip, spine, ribs, shoulder or wrist. The unfortunate part is that many a times steroid therapy is a necessary sin in the interest of the patient. The higher the dosage, greater is the damage. But experts are of the view that there is nothing like a safe dosage. Even pulse therapy is enough to cause damage. Steroids suppress collagen synthesis and delay wound healing too.

Treatment

i. Calcium supplement
ii. Vitamin D supplement
iii. Bisphosphonates
iv. Exercise
v. Stop or minimal dose of steroids consumption

If strict treatment protocol is adhered to combat steroid induced osteoporosis, the damage can be minimised to a great extent

Does Arthritis Lead to Osteoporosis?

Relationship

Yes, arthritis generally leads to osteoporosis because of sedentary lifestyle led by arthritic patients, although reverse is not true.

Generally the rheumatoid arthritis which strikes between 20 to 40 years debilitates the patient and the chronic inactivity owing to pain and swelling of joints makes proper walk and exercises difficult. This leads to osteoporosis of bones. Similarly in osteoarthritis patients (degenerative type) the joint problems reduce mobility of patient and ultimately osteoporosis sets in. Usually osteoarthritis develops in patients who are above 50 years.

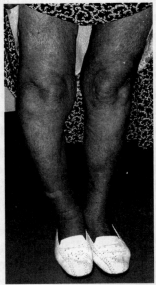

Fig. 3.6 Old arthritic patient

Remedy

i. Early detection, corrective steps and aggressive management of arthritis.
ii. Exercises schedule as per health status.
iii. Preventive anti osteoporotic treatment for risk patients in form of Calcium, Vitamin D and Bisphosphonates.
iv. Emphasis on correct nutrition.

Chapter 4
Falls and Fractures

Fracture due to a fall from a height without any serious road accident should be considered as osteoporotic fracture unless proved otherwise. 5 percent of the people require hospitalisation because of fractures. Certain factors which contribute towards having such a fracture are:

i. Arthritis
ii. Psychological ailments
iii. Visual impairment
iv. Weak muscles
v. Neurological diseases disturbing the motion and balance
vi. Hearing and cognitive problems
vii. Slippery surface or obstacles in house
viii. Alcohol
xi. Urinary urgency (Prostrate hypertrophy)
x. Sedatives or medicines

History of previous fracture and insufficient activity are the two things usually predisposing senior citizens to fall.

The statistics shows that 33 percent of senior citizens actually fall every year but only 5 percent of them sustain a fracture. Many of the factors mentioned above are correctable and modifiable.

So, it is advised that in the houses and work places, environment has to be improved in all aspects that is, to modify the health of human being first modify the surrounding by removing obstacles like loose mats, wires, cables and small furniture's etc.

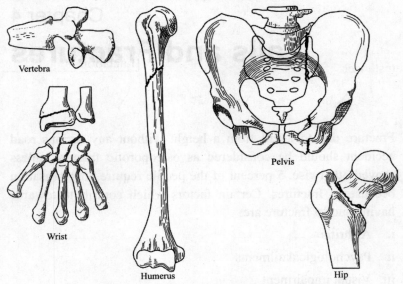

Fig. 4.1 Bone sites commonly involved in osteoporotic fractures

The commonest fracture sites are neck of femur, hip, lower end of the radius at the wrist, upper end of the humerus at the shoulder, vertebrae in the spinal column and ribs in the chest.

There is no national database of fracture prevalence in India and generally we presume it to be like those among Caucasians (American subcontinent):

- Proximal femur (18%)
- Vertebral column (16%)
- Distal radius (15%)
- Other locations (40%)

Fracture of Femur

- Intertrochanteric
- Neck of femur
- Sub capital (Type of fracture Neck of femur)

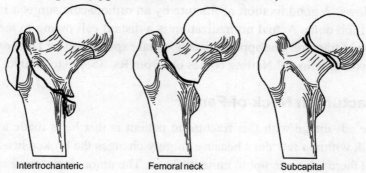

Fig. 4.2 Types of femoral fractures

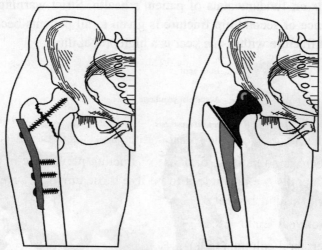

Fig. 4.3 Surgical repair of hip fractures

Intertrochantric fracture

Unites with a plate or nail. Dynamic hip screw plate system needed for fixation. Proximal Femoral Nailing (PFN) is the other option.

Surgery takes about one to two hours and fixation with modern implants is good and predictable. The hospital stay is 4-5 days followed by few months of recuperation at home. The patient has to walk without bearing weight during initial few weeks with the help of a walker, then partial and ultimately full weight bearing follows. A good fixation of fracture by an orthopaedic surgeon is half job done. Actual normalization is a distant call owing to the type of fracture. The approximate hospital expenditure for DHS or Proximal Femoral Nailing comes out from Rs. 35,000 to 70,000.

Fracture in Neck of Femur

The advantage with this fracture in patient is that he is made to walk within a few days because surgery changes the broken head and there is no attempt to unite the bone. The union is not tried in this fracture because of poor blood supply within this part of bone. The walker is used initially, later stick and then normal walk. All depends on fundamentals of patient's health. Strict warning for avoidance of second hip fracture is given to all patients because second fracture within one year is a high probability.

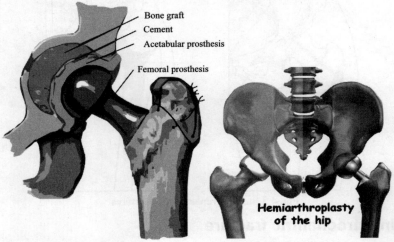

Fig. 4.4(a) Total Hip Replacement   Fig. 4.4(b) Partial Hip Replacement

Fracture in Lower end of the Radius at Wrist

Fracture in lower end of the radius at wrist is extremely common and mostly treated by closed reduction and plaster application but some times may need hospitalisation for external fixater/ distracter application in operation theatre when the fracture is invading the joint. The cost of surgery at wrist can be from Rs. 15,000 to 30,000.

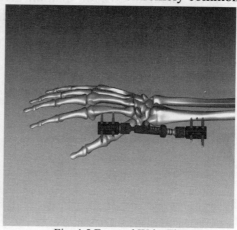

Fig. 4.5 External Wrist Fixator

Fracture at Proximal end of Humerus (at shoulder)

Requires close reduction and plaster but in some cases where fracture is in many pieces may need surgery in form of fixation by multiple wires, by buttress plate or changing of head of humerus all together (Hemiarthroplasty).

The shoulder is usually stiff following such fractures and needs a good amount of physiotherapy once

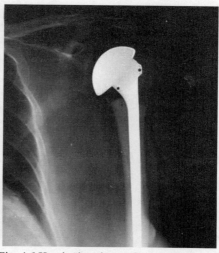

Fig. 4.6 Hemiarthroplasty of head of humerus

the fracture unites around six weeks later. Normally no plaster (POP) is needed and only shoulder arm immobiliser (Arm Pouch) is good enough. Cost of fixation at shoulder would be from Rs. 15,000–45,000. Changing of the head in Hemiarthroplasty with imported implant costs around Rs. 1.25–1.5 lakhs.

Chapter 5
Exercise and Bones

Exercise Helps Prevent Osteoporosis

Exercises help in making the bones strong by causing the muscles and tendons to pull on the bones, which in turn stimulates bone cells to produce more bone. In running or jogging, person's own body weight creates load on the bones or it can be done through dumbbells or gym machines. Our bones tend to fracture when we fall so the best way to protect from fall fractures is not to fall in the first place. Exercise not only helps in keeping bones healthy but it protects against fall and fractures as well improves balance and strength.

Exercise Builds Bones in Children

Reaching peak bone development at the age of 25-30 is possible provided exercises are an integral part of our life. That is why physical training in school fields and playgrounds in residential areas are of pivotal importance. A special emphasis on the strong requirement of young girls enjoying sports cannot be underplayed at this juncture because the bone tissue accumulated during the ages 11 to 13 approximately equals the amount lost during the 30 years following menopause. Ego Semen in Australia and other scientists in Europe have scientifically established this. In another study, boys who did more vigorous activity had 9 percent more bone area and 12 percent more bone strength than less active boys. Parents must discourage the 'Couch Potato Culture' in children. Here, there is a role for civic authorities who should provide playing areas in parks and not create impediments with their bizarre beauty ideas.

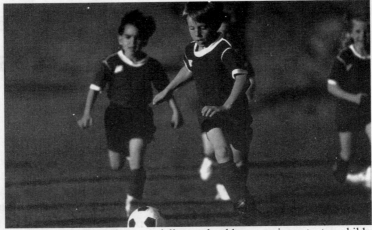

Fig. 5.1 Physical education especially at school becomes important, as children spend more time in front of the television and computer when home.

Exercise Maintains Bones in Adults

All of you can remember the pictures of US astronaut of Indian origin Sunita Williams working out on treadmill during her space travel. This is because weightlessness in the space makes the bones osteoporotic and it is easy to understand that in zero gravity muscles do not need to work as hard resulting in weakness. So for all of us on the earth the message is clear: exercises can build bones and muscles in youth and also maintain them later.

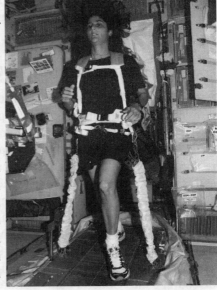

Fig. 5.2 Sunita Williams on Treadmill

Exercise Helps Bones of Elderly Too

Mehrsheed Sinaki and colleagues in USA and Japan found that when older post menopausal women used smaller weights to strengthen their back muscles over a period of two years, ten years down the road, they had stronger back muscles than their peers who did not exercise. Their bones were stronger too particularly their vertebrae and what is more important the exercises reduced the chance of getting fractures by almost three fold.

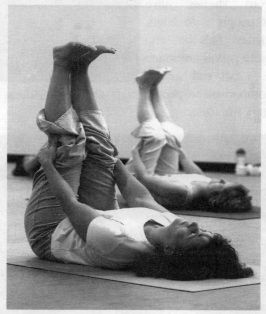

Fig. 5.3 Postmenopausal women, who took part in a two-year back exercise regimen, were half as likely to have wedged vertebrae as control patients.

Exercise helps posture and balance – prevents falls

Though a person with osteoporosis has a much greater risk of bone fracture than someone with normal bone mineral density, studies have shown that it is often a fall that causes the fracture. In fact every year two out of five (40 percent) people over sixty five fall at least once. So, avoiding falls could go a long way towards preventing fractures especially hip fractures.

Numerous studies have shown that people with better posture, better balance and greater muscle power are much less likely to fall and sustain injury in comparison to people with sedentary life style.

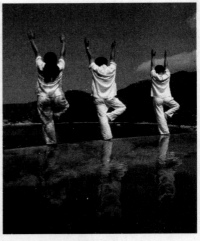

Fig. 5.4 Practice of Balance and Posture

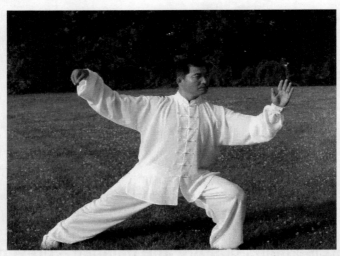

Fig. 5.5 Tai Chi is an ancient Chinese martial art consisting of a series of slow, gentle, continuous movements. It is particularly suitable for older people as it helps them to develop stronger muscles and better balance and concentration.

Women who sit for nine hours a day are more likely to have a hip fracture. Special muscle strengthening and training of balance program have reduced the risk of fall in elderly by 20-30 percent.

Exercise Your Bones

Regular weight bearing exercise helps build up bone mass in young people and helps maintain it in adults. Sports that involve lifting weights, running, sprinting, walking, jumping, skipping are good as also are dancing, playing hockey, cricket, tennis and field games. However the low impact exercises like swimming and cycling are beneficial for cardiovascular health and improving muscle strength but will not promote bone formation. If you have been out of touch from exercises for a long time, better start them gradually and progress over a period of time. Two short exercise sessions separated by eight hours is better than long sessions. Maintain balanced healthy diet along with exercises to prevent osteoporosis.

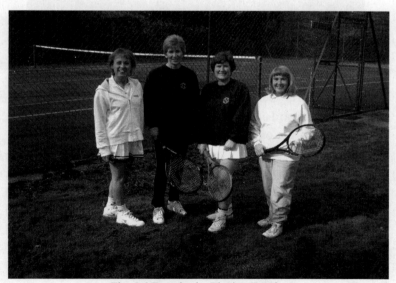

Fig. 5.6 Exercise by Playing Tennis

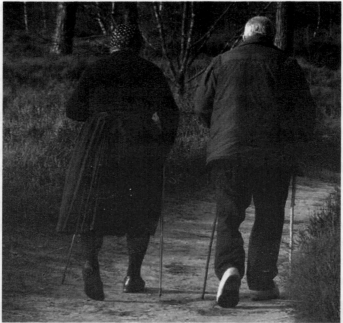
Fig. 5.7 Brisk Walking

Exercise Aids Rehabilitation

Chronic pain is perhaps most problematic in people with kyphosis (backward curvature of spine) this is the consequence of osteoporosis in the elderly. It usually causes loss of height, poor posture and a shift in the centre of gravity, thereby increasing risk of fall and fracture. By strengthening muscles in the back the spine can be brought more upright, help reduce the pain and improve quality of life. Exercises after fracture under supervision of physiotherapist are very important for regaining normal life and independence.

Don't over do it

Women and teenage girls who exercise to an extreme degree can develop amenorrhoea (cessation of menstruation) due to oestrogen deficiency. This deficiency contributes to bone loss.

Pre-occupation with excessive exercise may lead to eating disorders like anorexia or bulimia. The loss of essential nutrients in these conditions makes bones thin. Too much exercise can lead to stress fractures in legs and joint damage. Excessive exercise in osteoporotic elderly can lead to fractures. Exercise regimens should be tailored to each individual's own abilities and circumstances.

Tips: How not to Fall

- Keep the house, bathroom, and floor dry and use non-slippery material for floors
- Have a proper illumination within the house, always use night lamp in bedrooms
- Use hand railings on stairs and stick while walking liberally for support
- Get your eyesight checked regularly
- Remove any roadblocks in the house and surroundings like toys, stools, chairs, footwear, water pipes, wires etc., try and have as even a surface as possible in the residence
- Hip protection braces for individuals at high risk
- Using walker by shaky elderly suffering with neurological disorders is a good idea

Chapter 6
Nutrition

Calcium

Calcium is abundant in the body and most of it, about 99 percent, is deposited in the bones. Calcium has the most important role in preventing and treating osteoporosis. The best way to get calcium is by eating calcium rich foods. WHO advises 1000-1300 mg/day of Calcium intake but Indians on an average consume only 450 mg/day. While calcium alone cannot treat osteoporosis, it increases the effectiveness of total therapy. Calcium is also essential for functioning of heart, muscles, nerves and blood vessels. Whenever there is insufficient dietary calcium, bony calcium dissolves and goes back to bloodstream to maintain proper calcium level in the blood. So, if we take less calcium in food, bones will have to give out more. Calcium absorption in intestine may be reduced because of alcohol, excessive caffeine and phosphates from fizz drinks. Also high fat foods, antacids (medicine to reduce burning in stomach) and high fibre diet hinders absorption of calcium.

Calcium requirement of a person depends on age and sex.

Age Group	Calcium (mg/day)
0-6 months	300-400
7-12 months	400
1-3 years	500
4-6 years	600
7 to 9 years	700

10-18 years	1300
Women: 19 to menopause Men: 19-65 years	1000
Women: Post-menopause Men: 65 plus years	1300
Pregnancy	1200
Lactation	1000

(**Source:** FAO/WHO: Human Vitamin and Mineral requirement 2002)

During skeletal growth phase in children one can absorb 75 percent of ingested calcium while adults can absorb upto 30 percent only.

We should avoid taking more than 500 mg of calcium tablet daily unless and until advised more by the doctor.

Sources of Calcium and Vitamin D

Rich sources of calcium include milk, yoghurt, cheese, tofu, sardines, salmon, turnips and some green leafy vegetables, such as spinach, broccoli etc. The main sources of Vitamin D are cold saltwater fish, for example, salmon, halibut, herring and tuna; fortified milk; egg yolks; liver and fish oils. Some foods interfere with calcium availability. Excessive proteins, sodium and caffeine can increase the urinary excretion of calcium while excessive fibre can interfere with its absorption. Foods rich in oxalic acid (oxylates), such as spinach, rhubarb, beet greens and almonds and legumes such as beans and peas which are high in phytates, bind the calcium and make it unavailable.

Myth about Calcium

Myth that kidney will form stones because of calcium intake is baseless. Taken in right dosage there is nothing to worry.

Calcium carbonate is a less expensive form, and it provides highest elemental calcium but it causes constipation which is already a bothersome issue in the elderly. That is the reason why calcium citrate is preferred in old patients (easily absorbed).

Calcium may interfere with certain drugs like medicines for thyroid disorders, convulsions, steroids and antibiotics, so if you are taking any of these, take it separately.

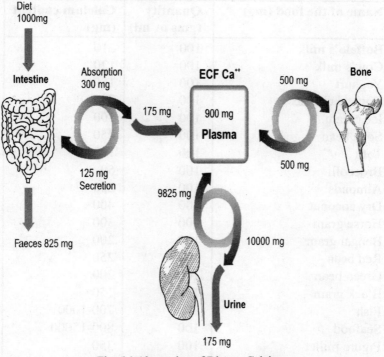

Fig. 6.1 Absorption of Dietary Calcium

Some seasonings and flavouring agents are high in clacium, but are generally used in a small quantity. Regular use of these ingredients in food preparation will, in the long run, increase the calcium content in the diet.

- Arrowroot flour
- Gingili seeds
- Poppy seeds
- Sunflower seeds

- Curry leaves
- Mustard seeds
- Cumin seeds
- Coriander
- Cloves
- Cardamom
- Lime peel
- Safflower seeds
- Fennel seeds
- Jaggery

Calcium Rich Foods

Name of the food (mg)	Quantity (gms or ml)	Calcium content (mg)
Buffalo's milk	100	210
Cow's milk	100	120
Yoghurt	100	150
Cottage cheese	100	790
Ice cream	100	100
Soya bean	100	250
Tofu	100	150
Broccolli	100	50
Almonds	100	230
Dry coconut	100	400
Horse gram	100	300
Bengal gram	100	200
Red bean	100	250
Green bean	100	200
Black gram	100	150
Fish	100	700-1000
Seafood	100	800-15000
Figure millet	100	350
Amaranth leaves	100	300-450
Cauliflower greens	100	630
Colocasia leaves	100	250-350
Knolkol greens	100	750
Carrot leaves	100	350
Turnip leaves	100	700

Dates	100	120
Raisin and Black currant	100	80
Wood apple	100	130
Egg	100	60
Tamarind	100	170
Walnut	100	80
Pistachio nut	100	140
Parsley	100	400
Mint	100	200
Coriander leaves	100	180

Recommended Calcium Allowance

Age group	Calcium (mg/day)
0-6 months	300-400
7-12 months	400
1-3 years	500
4-6 years	600
7-9 years	700
10-18 years	1300
Women: 19 - menopause Men: 19-65 years	1000
Women: Post-menopause Men: 65+years	1300
Pregnancy	1200
Lactation	1000

Vitamin D

Vitamin D is main regulator of calcium. It promotes absorption of calcium in intestine, decreases excretion of calcium from kidneys,

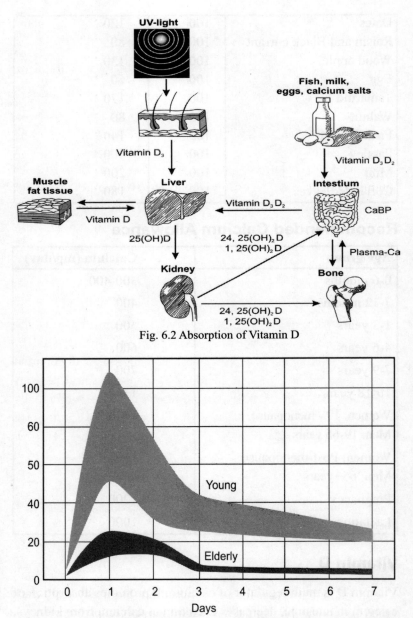

Fig. 6.2 Absorption of Vitamin D

Fig. 6.3 Serum concentration of Vitamin D (n mol/L) in Young and Elderly

helps maturation of bone cells and promotes incorporation in the bone and also reduces blood pressure. So if we take calcium without Vitamin D the calcium level in the blood is unlikely to be maintained. Sunlight is the biggest source of the Vitamin D, from skin to bloodstream then to liver and kidney, Vitamin D gets transformed into active forms.

India despite of having abundant sunlight has Vitamin D deficiency in almost all age groups – children, adults, pregnant women and elderly citizens. Studies show that 78% of Indians are Vitamin D deficient. The desired levels are 30 ng/ml in blood but most Indians have 4-12 ng/ml.

Deficiency of Vitamin D may be on account of less exposure to sunlight (minimum thirty minutes of exposure is required every day in good sunlight). Dark pigmentation of skin, sunscreen lotions, sunscreens films in the vehicle, fully covered cloths etc. are other reasons cited for lack of Vitamin D synthesis in Indians.

Vitamin D supplements are required for compensating the deficiency. Most experts recommend daily 400 to 1000 IU of Vitamin D. Native form of Vitamin D is considered good. Potential risk of excessive Vitamin D includes damage to central nervous system. Vitamin D metabolism is inhibited in patients with kidney and liver disorders, so the active form of Vitamin D is required for them. The dosage of active forms is:

- Alfa Calcidol—0.5-1 mcg/day orally
- Calcitriol—0.5 mcg/day orally

The inactive early form of Vitamin D is usually available with calcium tablets in the market.

Vitamin K

Vitamin K is important for bone formation. Normally leafy dark green vegetables like spinach, mustard leaves etc. provide it.

Bone Health	Quantity (gms)	Vitamin K Content (mcg)
Mustard leaves	100	138
Spinach	100	100
Okra (bhindi)	100	80
Radish leaves	100	260
Fenugreek leaves	100	400
Lotus stem	100	405

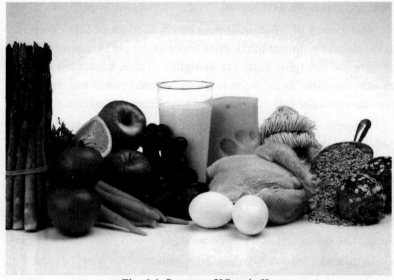

Fig. 6.4 Sources of Vitamin K

Chapter 7
Lifestyle

It is of utmost importance to modify and rectify certain lifestyle habits like avoiding to smoke, drink and excessive use of beverages. Keep disease under control. Get yourself periodically checked for early detection of diseases like Hypothyroidism, Diabetes, Epilepsy and digestive ailments.

Smoking

Smoking weakens bones and also damages heart and lungs. It has been scientifically established that prolonged smoking in males leads to osteoporosis. In females smoking precipitates menopause prematurely leading to lower oestrogen level. This hormone strengthens the bone, therefore smoking indirectly affects the female bones negatively. Smoking also reduces blood circulation to limbs and in case of fracture associated with wound, smoking delays wound healing definitely.

Alcohol

Regular alcohol consumption of more than 60 ml a day may result in osteoporosis in young men and women. Also, drinking affects the food intake and impedes food absorption in alimentary canal leading to calcium deficiency.

People with excessive alcohol consumption (>60 ml daily) have a 40 percent increased risk of sustaining an osteoporotic fracture compared to people with moderate or no alcohol intake. High intakes of alcohol cause secondary osteoporosis due to direct adverse effects on bone-forming cells, on the hormone that regulates calcium metabolism and deteriorating the nutritional status (calcium, protein and vitamin D deficiency).

Coffee

Caffeine has been shown to produce small amount of increase in urinary calcium excretion and small decrease in calcium absorption. Thus, it weakens the bones in the long run. Therefore, excessive intake of coffee should be avoided.

Carbonated drinks

Ca (Calcium) and Po_4 (Phosphate) have a balance in human body and because of excessive phosphate in carbonated drinks, the calcium absorption is reduced leading to deleterious affect on bones. Anyway they have hardly any nutritional value. Children are advised to avoid them. But ensuring easy availability of tasty health drinks is a challenging task and here the carbonated drinks have an edge. Certainly it is a welcome idea that schools and work places encourage healthy drinks and foods.

Beauty Pageants and Bones

'Well are these girls really beautiful?' asked Dr Veena, a senior physician, watching the ramp walk of skinny looking girls on Television. The same view was echoed by organisers of a beauty pageant in Amsterdam last year when they turned down a participant for low Body Mass Index(BMI).She was too thin to be called healthy.

The experts are of the opinion that the BMI of a young girl if less than 20 means that she is underweight and the bones are likely to become osteoporotic. The positive message is maintaining the body mass index is paramount and starving in young girls to look thin is an abhorrent idea.

IOF(International Osteoporosis Foundation) took an initiative and brought many former Beauty Queens of the world / universe on one platform in Bangkok 3 years ago. They appealed to all young girls of the world to eat well and not starve themselves. Real beauty lies in looking healthy and not emaciated. Thus, the desire to look extremely thin can be gravely dangerous.

In fact, parents, teachers, doctors and elders should ask the impressionable minded girls between 12 and 20 to shun dieting and drink milk, eat high protein diet, enjoy sports and exercise. These young girls are future mothers and obsession with that cachexic look is deplorable. Remember, a healthy body is not obese.

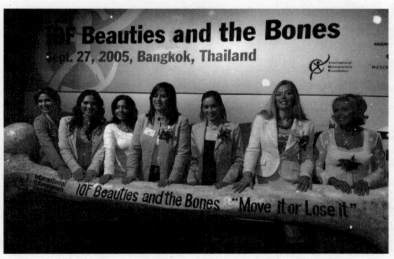

Chapter 8
The Treatment of Osteoporosis

The ultimate aim of treatment is to prevent fractures and the morbidity associated with it. Like we treat Hypertension to prevent Brain haemorrhages (strokes) and high blood sugar to prevent Diabetic retinopathy (eyes) and Nephropathy (kidney damage), similarly there is need to treat osteoporosis to prevent hip and other fractures because majority of fractures above 45 are due to osteoporosis. Weak bones give away with minimal trauma like a slip in bathroom, twist on stairs and fall in the home or park.

Treatment

i. Calcium and Vitamin D should be supplemented along with various other medicines given to treat osteoporosis.
ii. Bone building nutrition
iii. Exercise
iv. Treatment of pain
v. Anti Resorptive Therapy (therapy to reduce bone destruction – Bisphosphonates, Calcitonin, Raloxifene)
vi. Osteoanabolic therapy (therapy to build more bone - Fluoride anabolic steroids, Parathormone / PTH etc.)

vii. HRT (Hormone Replacement Therapy) for short periods in most cases.

Hormone Replacement Therapy

The loss of estrogen after menopause results in bone stock depletion and is maximum in first five years. The speed is slow after 7-8 years of menopause. Since menopause is a natural event in all women's life hormonal variation and its handling becomes crucial. The advantage is that HRT treatment not only helps fight osteoporosis but also treats certain women specific post-menopausal problems, like hot flushes, uneasiness, bodyache etc. HRT is generally used in immediate post menopausal women. The tablets cost Rs. 5-10 and are usually consumed on daily basis.

Side effects - mood swings, periodic vaginal bleeding and disturbance in menstrual cycles, hypertension and rarely cancer of uterus and breast. Due to these side effects oestrogen hormone or oestrogen – progesterone hormone combination is less used these days and hormone like medicines has taken greater role.

The testosterone **male hormone** increases bone density but prostatic hypertrophy is a side effect and has to be watched. In males the menopausal equivalent 'andropause' strikes much later, say at 60.

Anti Resorptive Therapy
Bisphosphonates

These deposit on surface of bone and reduce resorption of bone; whereas bone building is going on unhindered and thereby increasing bone density. The good thing is that bone remodeling is not stopped by these agents. In the west these agents are used for prevention and treatment both. Whereas in our country these agents are mainly used for treatment only. Generally bisphosphonates are effective in all types of osteoporosis and in a way the most important and time tested arsenal against osteoporosis. In india we have

• Risedronate	Weekly therapy
• Ibandronate	Monthly therapy
• Alendronate	Daily or weekly therapy

The one year treatment with oral Bisphosphonates costs about Rs. 1500 in India but may cost many times more in Europe and USA.

The above mentioned bisphosphonates are for oral intake.

I/V Ibandronic acid administered once in 3 months and I/V Zoledronic acid administered once in a year are intravenous methods of bisphosphonate administration.

Advantages of I/V Ibandronic acid is it can be given in non ambulatory patients like fracture patients. The cost of intravenous Ibandronic acid is around Rs. 5000 and that of Zoledronic acid around Rs. 3,000 to 15,000 depending upon company. But Zoledronic acid infusion needs one day hospitalisation.

Contraindications

- Breast feeding
- Pregnancy
- Relative contraindication — poor kidney function

Warning: All those women who want to conceive must stop bisphosphonates at least 6 to 12 months well in advance because this drug remains in blood circulation for a long time, which may be harmful.

Oral Bisphosphonates are poorly absorbed in presence of calcium and food so should be given empty stomach in morning. To see effectiveness of therapy; 3 months post commencement of treatment, bone markers can be checked for watching the improvement. The one year therapy is known for 50% reduction in vertebral, hip and other fractures. After six months even bone density can be checked to watch for improvement. There are a few new members about to join this family, Pamidronate and Lasofoxifene.

Safety Valve

It is understood that after prolonged bisphosphonate therapy of 2 to 5 yrs fracture risk reduces by 50% in hip and 89% in spine. There is no way to guarantee 100% risk reduction. Bone density increases but usually doesn't normalise.

SERMS – (Selective Estrogen Receptor Modifying drugs)

Raloxifene 60 mg taken daily by post menopausal women for 1 year increases bone density by 2-3 percent thereby decreasing fracture risk by 30-50 percent. Even those who go for hormone therapy are gradually shifted to SERMS.

The selective oestrogen receptor modulator drugs are inexpensive and are effective. It also helps in decreasing risk of breast cancer, very effective between 55-65 years of age. It has been also tried in men but results are not clearly known.

Osteoanabolic therapy
Anabolic Steroids

Anabolic steroids are also injected at 3-4 weekly intervals in elderly patients and they increase muscle mass and some bone stock too. These steroids are generally used (rather misused) by various sportsmen as body building and performance enhancing agents. They also have side effects and a long term use in elderly is avoided. The injection costs only Rs. 50-100 in Indian currency and no hospitalisation is required, it is just an outpatient procedure. There are a few recent reports attributing minor anabolic action to bisphosphonates.

Bone Forming Agents
Parathormone or Teriparatide (PTH)

Earlier discussed drugs are only inhibiting bone resorption and what we badly need now are agents which can form bone what we call osteoanabolic or osteoblastic agents technically. PTH is a hormone, a polypeptide (Protein group). PTH infact promotes Calcium transport into alimentary canal and helps synthesis of active Vitamin D in kidney. More deeply, it increases life of bone forming cells osteoblasts in body and helps in collagen synthesis (the protein matrix of bone), but Ca and Vit. D is must along with PTH to improve bone density in real means. Studies have shown that PTH therapy for 1-2 years in the form of injections increases bone density by 10-30percent thereby decreasing fracture risk up to 65 percent. So with PTH injectable therapy, the fracture risk reduction is maximum but the limiting factors of this therapy are daily injections and exorbitant cost. Although the subcutaneous injections are administered easily by the patient him/herself or family.

- Forteo- Ili Lilly-18 month therapy - Rs. 2 lakhs
- Bonista Ranbaxy - Rs. 1.80 Lakhs

The problem area is that daily injectable prefilled syringes are only reimbursed for central government employees (CGHS scheme) not by Insurance Co. generally. Even the CGHS employees are provided for after the first fracture plus, DEXA scan proved cases of osteoporosis.

PTH has no synergistic action with Bisphosphonate, so it has to be taken solo. In our country expensive PTH is recommended for selected cases like:

i. Patients who sustained fracture inspite of being on bisphosphonate therapy.

ii. Patients who do not show any increase in BMD after bisphosphonate, HRT and SERM therapy.

iii. Severe osteoporosis cases with history of first fracture sustained. In such cases aim is to prevent second fracture. The patient has to be on PTH therapy for 18 to 24 months followed by bisphosphonate therapy for a maximum period of 5 years. The big challenge before the medical fraternity is how to manage osteoporosis patient if the life is long. The science is yet to come out with a therapy which can effectively check disease 10 to12 years after the commencement of treatment.

Strontium

Strontium is also an agent which has bone forming action and helps in Osteoporosis treatment. Strontium Ranelate tablets are taken orally and are available in India. Taken over a period of 6 months, improves bone density but the quality of bone is not as good as with PTH, therefore is considered a second class treatment. Therapy is cheap and a 2gm tablet/day is costing just Rs. 50- 75 in India.

There are many other agents undergoing human trials and research. Tibolone is one such drug but has not taken off because of observed side effects.

Calcitonin

Calcitonin is a polypeptide (protein) hormone produced by thyroid gland in body. It reduces resorption of bone and has very potent action on vertebral column. It is used more for reducing pain and less for improving bone density. In India it is used in nasal spray form, which is sniffed everyday through alternate nostrils. One pack has 30 doses. Occasionally irritation in nose and nausea /

vomiting has been reported but not frequently. It may be used during pregnancy and breast feeding. The 30 dose aerosol pack costs about Rs. 1000 in India. The therapy has to be continued for at least 3-6 months for desirable effects.

Fluorides

It is also a bone forming agent but it is not preferred in India and many other countries because of poor quality of bone production and side effects.

Growth hormones

Growth hormones have an anabolic action, generally in children but have to be monitored intensely.

Isoflavones and Phytoestrogens

Isoflavones function primarily to suppress bone resorbtion by stimulating bone cell growth and differentiation. Given in doses of 400 – 600 mg/day, they are useful in both young post menopausal women with a high bone turn over and elderly women with established osteoporosis. Phytoestrogens are plant compounds with estrogenic biological actions. Used mainly in patients who can not tolerate estrogen as a part of the Hormone Replacement Therapy. It is mainly seen in soy containing foods. 45 gm of soy flour or 60 gm of soy proteins per day is the recommended dosage. Both are still in experimental stages.

Assessment of Risk fracture

- One minute risk test by IOF FRAX tool, created by WHO can give you an idea how you will do in the coming 10 years
- BMD
- BMI
- Risk Factors

Role of Surgery in Osteoporotic Spine Fracture

Should we avoid it

Fractures of spine without any neurological involvement, that is, where bladder and bowel functions are normal, patient can comfortably urinate and defaecate, there is no weakness or numbness in the limbs, such patients do not require any spinal fixation. All they require is rest and painkillers for a period of minimum 6 to 12 weeks. Mostly such patients have minimal compression of vertebra and usually at a single level.

In cases of gross compression fractures where the height of vertebrae is reduced by half, a special treatment called vertebroplasty (injections of bone cement into the vertebrae under the image intensifier (TV control)) a can be done. The procedure requires PMMA bone cement and special disposable infiltration set. In recent advances, balloon kyphoplasty (instead of bone

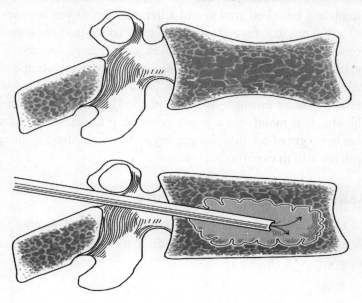

cement a balloon is inflated in the vertebrae) is also done. This procedure is more expensive than earlier one. A CT scan of spine is a must before going for vertebroplasty and proper assessment is required to avoid complications. The usual cost of vertebroplasty is Rs. 40 to 70 thousand in private hospitals. Procedure if done properly gives good relief from backache immediately.

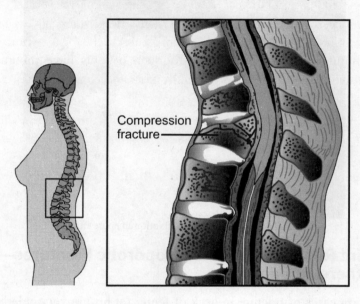

Spinal fixation in cases of neurological involvement is done generally in the form of pedicle screws and rods system. The cost of surgery is usually from Rs.60 thousand to 100 thousand. The surgery does not guarantee improvement in weakness and numbness. It is mainly to reduce compression on nerves, stabilize the spine and proper nursing care of patient.

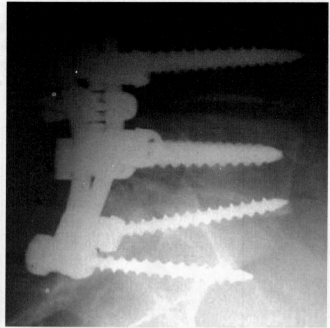

Fig. 8.1 Pedicle screw and rod fixation in spine fracture

Joint Replacement in Osteoporotic Fractures—Is there a need?

Yes, in cases of fracture in neck of femur (at hip) in very elderly people, changing the head of femur (ball at the top) alone, what is called as Hemiarthroplasty, may not be a long-term solution. As the person walks, the metal ball rubs on the acetabulam (the roof socket) making the hip painful. Obviously a painful hip is not compatible with long and active lifespan. So now most of the surgeons in east and west are resorting to total hip replacement (the ball and socket both) instead of hemi replacement (broken ball of hip only).

One of the important factors is the expenditure of such a surgery. Average expenditure incurred on bipolar (ball only) replacement is Rs. 35 to 80 thousand and for cemented Total Hip

Replacement it is from Rs. 60 to 100 thousand. The rates are not for 5 star hospitals.

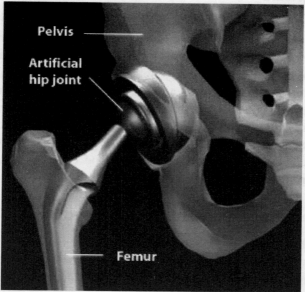

Fig. 8.2 Total hip replacement

Note: The wide range of expenses is on account of implant being Indian or Imported.

The choice of THR is between cemented and un-cemented. Cemented hip is less expensive but is generally used for patients above 65 who are unlikely to require revision in hip replacement in their lifetime.

The un-cemented hip is a choice for patient above 45-50 because they are likely to need revision of ball and socket 15 to 20 years later. The removal of the cement from the bone during revision surgery is a problematic undertaking and is therefore avoided whenever possible. The implant of uncemented hip is costlier by Rs. 30 to 40 thousand. There are Indian implants in replacement surgery too but unlike trauma implants (plates, nails, screws) artificial joint market is still ruled by overseas multinational companies like Johnson & Johnson, Zimmer, Smiths Nephew, Stryker to name a few.

What Bothers Patients about Government Hospitals

Whatever is the claim of the Government hospitals, the fact is the cost of treatment accrued here is just 50 percent less in comparison to private hospitals. The reality is, the implants and medicines for the patients are generally not provided in these institutions. Needless to say that time is a big casualty in these institutions and patients cannot exercise the choice of specialist which leads to a sense of insecurity. Besides this, the impersonal care, crowded atmosphere and not so pleasing services in such a set up of India make it less popular although there is no clear evidence about compromise in quality of actual treatment.

The Reimbursement Scene in India

Reimbursement for the health check-ups in Indian scenario is almost non-existent except in few public sector concerns and in semi government setups. Usually check-ups are allowed by institutions that have their hospitals or less expensive arrangements with government hospitals.

The insurance companies who provide cashless health insurance policy called 'mediclaim' do not reimburse osteoporosis investigations and BMD screening. They do provide reimbursement for fractures provided it needs hospitalisation. It usually happens in case of hip fractures, less often in wrist, shoulder and spine fractures. In the present scenario other than hip fracture, where hospitalisation is a must, the patients have to pay for the treatment on their own. The other disappointing factor is denial of insurance coverage by companies to people above 55. It is almost an unwritten rule.

After the first fracture the reimbursement covers only the fracture treatment up to 3 months. There is no coverage for the long-term osteoporosis treatment even when his or her bone mineral densitometry test proves it. In various countries of

Asia pacific like Australia, Japan, Hong Kong and Thailand osteoporosis treatment after the first fracture is reimbursed. The reality is that osteoporosis treatment after the first fracture is in the interest of the insurance company too in order to avoid second fracture. The statistics shows that 70 to 80 percent people sustain second fracture within one year of the first fracture, naturally the management is more expensive then prevention. But the insurance companies are happy being 'Penny Wise, Pound Foolish'.

AFI advises all those people who can afford to go in for mediclaim policy of at least Rs. 100 to 200 thousand if the person is less than 40 and Rs. 300 to 400 thousand in case the person is above 40. Mediclaim policy is all the more important if they enjoy no health facility from CGHS, State Government, Public Sector, and Corporate Sectors. The Government of India has devised an insurance policy for poor people (Below Poverty Line) because expenditure on health is one of the biggest reasons of indebtedness in this class. Obviously this class whether urban or rural lacks both reserves and planning. The penetration and success of this scheme is yet to be assessed. A civilized society should always dutifully stand for its not so well to do section.

Chapter 9
Bone Health in School Children

Nightmarish Deformities in Children: Rickets

Calcium and Vitamin D deficiency leads to weakening of long bones in children. The disease is called Rickets, at initial stage prominence of forehead, broadening of bones at wrists and knees are noticed. Later the bones bend inwards at the knees or outwards leading to deformed legs and extreme difficulty in walking. The deformity of bowing of legs internally in children is called Genu Varus and external bending is called Genu Valgus. If corrected at an early stage, medicinal treatment plus splintage to support the legs is sufficient but severe deformities need surgical corrections. Generally if left untreated up to 7-8 years of age surgical intervention is almost a rule.

The heavy doses (in form of tablets, powder, injections) of calcium and vitamin D is given to the child for a sustained period along with good massage of Vitamin D oil followed by 40 minutes sunbath daily. The supporting splints and corrective shoes also benefit a lot. Rickets not only disables the child at a very playful age but also afflicts the child psychologically with depression, poor academic performance and low self esteem.

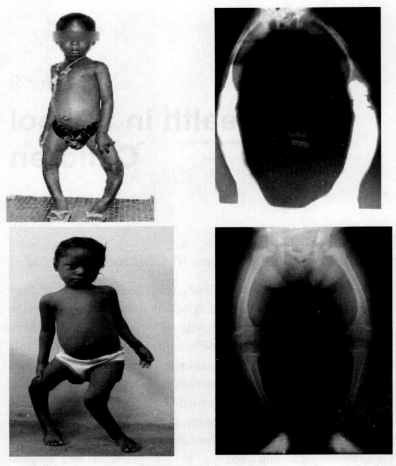

Fig. 9.1 Rickets

Surgical intervention is in the form of correcting the alignment of bones by osteotomising the long bone (cutting the bone and making it straight), and further the union of bone will need a plaster for 2-3 month. Generally the results are good but it is advisable to treat calcium and Vitamin D deficiency preferably before deformity sets in and for those who miss the bus at least should correct deficiency after the surgery.

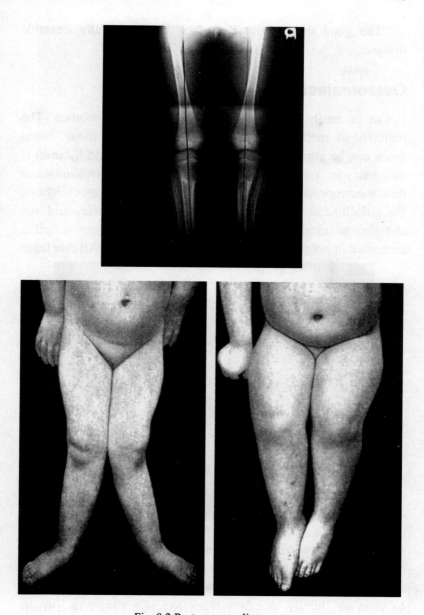

Fig. 9.2 Post surgery alignment

The good thing about Rickets is that it is fully treatable disease.

Osteomalacia

It can be easily called as the menace of young women. The majority of mothers-in-law and daughters-in-law (Saas, bahu) feuds can be attributed to osteomalacia. Calcium and Vitamin D deficiency in young women is called osteomalacia. Osteomalacia unlike osteoporosis is a painful condition. Right from childhood the girl child in India is discriminated vis-à-vis male child and therefore her nutrition suffers a great deal. The deficiency is further increased in pregnancy and then in lactation phase. All this leads

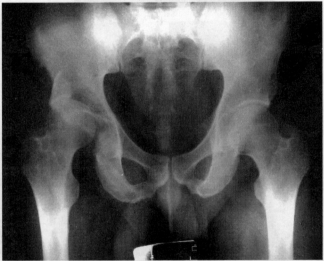

Fig. 9.3 Osteomalacia

to osteomalacia and if Calcium and Vitamin D is not compensated fully the pain in spine and pelvic bones mainly makes her almost unfit for rigorous domestic chores. When the young woman fails to cope up, family members think she is malingering, so the family feuds begin. If the problem is treated with a good amount of Calcium and Vitamin D in a few weeks time the loss can be recovered. In these women bones at the hips and spine show looser zones visible on x-rays, but unlike osteoporosis, osteomalacia can be treated effectively in much shorter period. In addition to osteomalacia, woman may develop osteoporosis then truly and mostly they may be labelled as osteoporomalacia.

Women reach their peak bone mass at the age of 30 and after that they lose bone mass. Good nutrition and sun exposure are of great help for rickets and osteomalacia.

Should Milk be Part of Mid Day Meal Programme in Schools?

The Mid-Day meal programme is an excellent means to provide food to children in schools. It serves a dual purpose ,first, improves nutrition, second it enhances the attendance in school. The debate is about the addition of milk, about 300ml, as part of the meals.

Milk is an essential part of the meal and has a pivotal role in bone building. If we as a country aspire to have people with strong bones it is mandatory to start the process right in the childhood, that is, schools. This is because the peak bone mass has to be attained at 25 to 30 and for that this time of childhood is very important. Scientific fact is, a girl child deposits enough bone between 11 and 14 which she is going to lose in between 45 and 60. Bones function like banks. Millions of children can't afford milk at all, getting 300 ml. of milk daily in school is going to tremendously boost their health. This is an investment for the future of our nation. The central government should join hands with state governments and realise this goal. India being the highest producer of milk in the world, the target is achievable.

The Issue of Lactose Intolerance is Over Played

The percentage is very nominal in children, little more in adults. The children who cannot tolerate milk can have milk in the form of rice and milk pudding, porridge, custard and curd. Same is true for adults. There is presumably a vested interest in underpinning the importance of milk in the life of growing children especially in a largely vegetarian country like India, so the government of India should add milk or milk products in children's diet at mid-day meal distribution in schools. It may increase the cost of mid-day meal programme, but in the long run it will be cost effective and worth the extra expenditure.

Balanced Diets for old people are given in Tables 10.1 and 10.2

Table 10.1 Balanced Diets (g) at High cost for Old People over 60 Years

Food stuff	Sedentary work			
	Males		Females	
	Veg	NVeg	Veg	NVeg
Cereals	320	320	220	220
Pulses	50	30	40	25
Green leafy vegetables	100	100	125	125
Other vegetables	75	75	75	75
Roots and tubers	75	75	50	50
Fruits	150	150	150	150
Milk	800	600	800	600
Fats and oils	30	30	30	30
Cheese	50	-	50	-
Meat and fish	-	100	-	100
Eggs	-	40	-	40
Sugar and jaggery	30	30	30	30

Table 10.2 Balanced Diets (g) at Moderate Cost for Old People over 60 Years

Food stuff	Sedentary work			
	Males		Females	
	Veg	NVeg	Veg	NVeg
Cereals	320	320	220	220
Pulses	70	55	60	45
Green leafy vegetables	100	100	125	125
Other vegetables	75	75	75	75
Roots and tubers	75	75	50	50
Fruits	75	75	75	75
Milk	600	400	600	400
Fats and oils	30	30	30	30
Meat and fish	-	60	-	60
Eggs	-	30	-	30
Sugar and jaggery	30	30	30	30
Multivitamin-mineral tablet	1	1	1	1

Table 10.3 Chemical Composition of Different Types of Cheese (Values per 100 g)

Cheese type	Moisture (g)	Calories (Kcal)	Protein (g)	Fat (g)	Carbohydrates total(g)	Ash (g)	Calcium (mg)	Phosphorus (mg)	Iron (mg)	Vitamin A (I.U.)	Thiamine (mg)	Riboflavin (mg)
Hard:												
Ceddar	37.0	398	25.0	32.2	2.1	3.7	750	478	1.0	1310	0.03	0.46
Swiss	39.0	370	27.5	28.0	1.7	3.8	925	563	0.9	1140	0.01	0.40
Semi-hard:												
Brick	41.0	370	22.2	30.5	1.9	4.4	730	455	0.9	1240	-	0.45
Roquefort	40.0	368	21.5	30.5	2.0	6.0	315	339	0.5	1240	0.03	0.61
Soft:												
Cottage (creamed)	78.3	106	13.6	4.2	2.9	1.0	94	152	0.3	170	0.03	0.25
Cottage (uncreamed)	79.0	86	17.0	0.3	2.7	1.0	90	175	0.4	10	0.03	0.28
Cream	51.0	374	8.0	37.7	2.1	1.2	62	95	0.2	1540	0.02	0.24
Camembert	52.2	299	17.5	24.7	1.8	3.8	105	184	0.5	1010	0.04	0.75
Lamburger	45.0	345	21.2	28.0	2.2	3.6	590	393	0.6	1140	0.06	0.50

Table 10.4 Chemical Composition of Whole Egg, Egg Yolk, White and Egg Powder (Values per 100 g)

Type	Moisture (g)	Protein (g)	Fat (g)	Carbohydrates (g)	Calories (kcal)	Ash (g)	Calcium (mg)	Phospherus (mg)	Iron (mg)	Vitamin A (I.U.)	Thiamine (mg)	Riboflavin (mg)	Niacin (mg)
Egg Hen													
Whole (without shell)	73.7	12.9	11.5	0.9	163	1.0	54	205	2.3	1180	0.11	0.30	0.1
Yolk	51.1	16.0	30.0	0.6	348	1.7	141	569	5.5	1400	0.22	0.44	0.1
White	87.6	10.9	trace	0.8	51	0.7	9	15	0.1	0	trace	0.27	0.1
Duck egg													
Whole (without shell)	70.4	13.3	14.5	0.7	196	1.1	56	195	2.8	1230	0.18	0.30	0.1
Goose egg													
Whole (without shell)	70.4	13.9	13.3	1.3	185	1.1	-	-	-	-	-	-	-
Turkey egg													
Whole (without shell)	72.6	13.1	11.8	1.7	170	0.8	-	-	-	-	-	-	-
Egg Hen													
Whole dried	2.0	48.9	42.9	2.5	509	3.7	194	832	9.0	4450	0.34	1.25	0.7
Egg white (powder)	8.8	80.3	0.2	5.7	37.2	5.1	66	110	1.0	0	0.04	1.99	0.2

Table 10.5 The Nutritive Value of Some Beverages (Values per 100 g)

Name of	Water (g)	Fat (g)	Total Carbohy-drates (g)	Calcium (mg)	Iron (mg)	Carotene (Pro-vitamin A) (ug)	Thiamine (mg)	Riboflavin (mg)	Vitamin C (mg)	Calorific value (Kcal)
Fruit juice										
Apple juice	85.9	-	13.8	6	0.5	4	0.02	0.02	1	53
Grape juice	85.3	-	13.7	8	0.3	20	0.02	0.02	3	55
Mango juice	84.2	-	14.6	12	0.5	1500	0.03	0.02	49	44
Orange juice	87.5	-	11.0	19	0.2	190	0.03	0.02	49	44
Pineapple juice	86.2	-	13.0	15	0.5	80	0.03	0.02	19	52
Tomato juice	93.5	-	4.3	7	0.4	1050	0.03	0.02	16	17
Dilute squash										
Orange squash	83.2	-	15.2	5	0.2	20	0.01	0.01	6	61
Lemon squash	83.4	-	15.0	7	0.2	-	0.01	0.01	5	60
Pineapple squash	82.9	-	15.2	6	0.2	50	0.01	0.01	5	61
Mango squash	82.9	-	15.6	8	0.2	500	0.01	0.01	6	62
Misceleneous beverages										
Coconut water	93.9	-	5.9	10	0.1	-	0.01	0.01	2	24
Coconut milk	89.8	7.2	2.0	20	0.2	-	0.02	0.01	1	76
Neera (sweet toddy)	84.7	-	14.3	40	1.0	-	0.02	0.02	13	57
Soft drinks, carbonated cold and ether sweet drinks	88.0	-	12.0	-	-	-	-	-	-	48
Sugarcane juice	90.2	-	9.1	10	1.1	-	0.02	0.02	5	36

Table 10.6 The Nutiritve Value of Vegetables and Fruits (Range of Values per 100g)

Nutrient	Green leafy vegetables	Roots and tubers	Other vegetables	Fruits
Moisture (g)	79-92	69-91	72-96	75-90
Calories (Kcal)	32-96	20-160	14-104	10-50
Carbohydrates (g)	4-14	4-38	4-20	2-20
Protein (g)	1.9-6.7	0.7-3.0	0.4-7.0	0.2-2.0
Fat (g)	0.1-1.7	0.1-0.3	0.1-0.1	0.1
Calcium (mg)	30-500	10-50	10-130	5-40
Iron (mg)	0.8-10.0	0.4-2.1	0.5-5.8	0.1-1.0
Carotene (µg)	1200-7500	30-3000	5-200	5-500
Ascorbic acid (mg)	48-220	3-24	2-66	2-700
Thiamine (mg)	0.05-0.10	0.05-0.10	0.04-0.25	0.05-0.2
Riboflavin (mg)	0.11-0.14	0.01-0.07	0.01-0.08	0.02-0.1
Nicotinic acid (mg)	0.1-0.8	0.3-1.2	0.2-0.9	0.2-0.4
Folic acid (mg)	10-20	3-6	5-10	6-9
Potassium (mg)	250-570	200-370	200-400	66-250
Sodium (mg)	4-91	18-60	10-45	5-15

Chapter 10
The Value of Milk

Milk has many nutrients and it comes from cows/buffalo. Cow's milk can be broken down into 7 major components

Cow milk (whole)		Buffalo milk (whole)	
Nutritional value per 100 g (3.5 oz)		Nutritional value per 100 g (3.5 oz)	
Energy	60 kcal		250 kJ
Carbohydrates	5.2 g		4.9 g
Sugars	5.2 g		4.9 g
Lactose	5.2 g		4.9 g
Fat	3.25 g		8.0 g
Saturated	1.9 g		4.2 g
Monounsaturated	0.8 g		1.7 g
Polyunsaturated	0.2 g		0.2 g
Protein	3.2 g		4.5 g
Water	88 g		81.1 g
Vitamin A equiv. 28 µg 3%		Calcium 195 mg	
Thiamine (Vit. B1) 0.04 mg 3%			
Riboflavin (Vit. B2) 0.18 mg 12%			

Vitamin B12 0.44 µg 18%
Vitamin D 40 IU 20%
Magnesium 10 mg 3%
Potassium 143 mg 3%
100 ml corresponds to 103 gm

Cow's milk

Contains, on average, 3.4% protein, 3.6% fat, 4.6% lactose, 0.7% minerals and supplies 66 kcal of energy per 100 grams.

Water

Cow milk boasts approximately 88% water. Cow's milk contains roughly 3% to 4% protein, of which about 80% is casein and 20% is whey.

Fat

Naturally, the fat content of cow's milk can range from 3% to 6%. In the United States, whole milk must contain at least 3.25% fat, while 2%, 1% and 0.5% of milk fat are regulated for reduced fat, low fat and skim varieties respectively. This doesn't sound too bad, but the fat content is actually much higher than we perceive. These percentages are by weight, not calories. This means that the 88% water is not only diluting the milk itself, but also the percentage of fat. Whole milk derives 50% of its calories from fat, 2% gets 35% of its calories from fat; 1% weighs in with 23% of its calories from fat and skimmed milk is the lone lightweight with 5% of calories from fat. People can drink milk freely for bones and those with heart problems can go for low fat milk.

Carbohydrate

When it comes to fibre and complex carbohydrates, milk is not a contender. It contains sugar, lactose to be specific. Approximately 5% of milk is sugar and not the fun sweet kind either. Lactose is known to create lactose intolerance in some people.

Water soluble Vitamins

Natural milk contains a fair amount of the C and B Vitamins. However, part of Vitamin C is weakened or destroyed during pasteurisation. It is believed that about 38% of the Vitamin B is also destroyed during pasteurisation.

Fat soluble Vitamins

Cow's milk contains Vitamins A, D, E, and a very small amount of K.

Minerals

The primary minerals in milk are Phosphorus and Calcium. The body needs to maintain a perfect balance of Phosphorus and Calcium. When too much of one is present, it depletes the other. That is why it is advisable to cut off the soft drinks and processed foods. Unfortunately, westernised diets are often loaded with phosphorus in the form of carbonated beverages and processed foods. Loss of soluble calcium, due to repeated boiling and pasteurisation, has now been recognised as a very important factor in growth and development of children, not only in the formation of bones and teeth, but also in the Calcium content of the blood. To strike a good balance, as far as sterilisation and maintenance of healthy components in milk is concerned, Ultra High Temperature (UHT) milk claims to be a scientifically viable concept .

UHT Milk

Fraudulent practices by unscrupulous milk vendors have led to adulteration of various types and magnitude resulting in the change of the nutrient content and volume of milk in order to earn profit.

In India, a large part of the population still buys unpasteurised raw milk which is mostly delivered daily by local milkman carrying bulk quantities in a possibly contaminated metal / aluminum containers which can harbour harmful bacteria and carries potential risk of food born diseases. Even the process of milking is unhygienic and cows are kept in poor sanitary conditions. Antibiotics and local medication given to the cows when they are sick changes the composition and could be harmful for human consumption.

A good substitute can be milk which is aseptically packaged and treated with Ultra High Temperature (UHT) available in Tetra Pak packages. This milk can be kept up to 4-6 months without refrigeration, does not need to be boiled after purchase. UHT technique boasts completely sterile process of giving milk a longer and safer shelf life by removing any harmful bacteria present in milk without adding any preservatives and without losing out on the essential nutrients required for a healthy living. UHT milk goes through a flash heating process, in which milk is heated at high temperature for a fraction of a second and cooled in sterile conditions, thus ensuring that all harmful bacteria is eliminated.

It is due to the flash heating, the milk can be consumed directly without boiling. After this process, milk is packed in a six layered Tetra Pak packaging, untouched by hand. The Tetra Pak package is made of four layers of food grade polyethylene, one layer of paper and one of aluminum foil, ensuring that the milk is protected from light, moisture and any bacteria. These packages are tamper evident (if carton packages are tampered with, they become puffy – indicating that they should not be consumed). Most importantly, milk in Tetra Pak packages can be stored for 4-6 months ambient temperature without refrigeration and they do not contain any preservatives.

Since milk is an essential supplement of Indian vegetarian diet, we need to ensure its purity and safety in addition to nutritional adequacy; essentially and adequately labeled for consumer interest and nutritionally protected.

There is no doubt that this tetrapak milk is consumed well in west but in India people will take time to get convinced.

Chapter 11
Bone Health at Work Place

Bone health at work place programme is a unique initiative of its style taken by Arthritis Foundation of India in NCR. Basically maintaining the bone health is the responsibility of the individuals but the management of the company and institutions can also help them by providing them right kind of environment. It is a straightforward case of good health (for workers) means good economics (for institution). If the staff is healthy the efficiency and production is bound to increase and the medical bills are bound to decrease. In essence every organisation should try and be a 'Bone-responsible organisation'. It is anergonomic concept too.

Action-line

i. Every one should take IOF one minute risk test and assess the risk. (see p. 3)
ii. All men/women having risk factor should go in for BMD test.
iii. All women above 40 and all men above 50 should go in for the BMD test. (see p. 25)

iv. A gymnasium space for exercise is to be provided where some equipment for workout and relaxation exercises are available.

v. The employees should learn the art of utilising 15 min from their lunch hour or coffee-break for having workouts in the gymnasium.

vi. The canteen should be asked to provide bone healthy products for refreshment and not (carbonated beverages). Encourage juices, salted butter milk, flavoured milk, nuts, fruits, sweet butter milk, low fat protein biscuits etc.

vii. Educate employees about bone health.

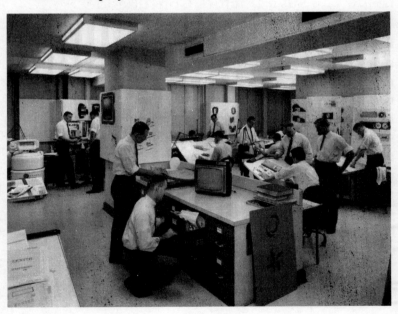

Chapter 12
OTC Drugs

Helps you save Doctors Consultation

The minimal levels of pain, swelling in musculoskeletal disorders, osteomalacia and micro fractures of osteoporosis can be handled by patients on their own with the help of 'over the counter' (OTC) medicines. These medicines can be bought from medical stores without doctor's prescriptions. No doubt patients will save on doctor's fees. Nevertheless, one shouldn't overdo it, especially when diagnosis is not clear and problem is sustained for a longer time. In a nutshell, OTC products help you self medicate, save time and money both, but reasonable judgement should be exercised. There are numerous brands of drugs available in the market.

List of Medicines (Can be used as and when required)

Painkillers	Price
i. Tb Crocin Pain relief	
ii. Tb Disprin (Glaxo)	
iii. Tb Crocin (Glaxo)	
iv. Tb Anacin	Rs. 2-3 /tablet
v. Tb Saridon (Denzon)	

| vi. Tb Combiflam (Aventis) | |
| vii. Diclovin Plus (Wings Pharma) | |

Local Ointments

i. Volini Gel (Ranbaxy)	
ii. Medicreme	Rs. 30 to 45 /tube
iii. Iodex	

Ca/Vit D Preparations (One per day to supplement deficit in diet)

i. Calcium Sandoz for Women and Children	Rs. 3 to 6 / tablet

Antacids (To reduce burning and acidity in stomach)

i. Tb Digene	
ii. Digene Syrup	Rs. 2-4 / tab
iii. Tb Zinetac	

Antioxidants (For Rejuvenation of body)

i. Tb Revital	
ii. Tb Antoxid	Rs. 10-20 / tab
iii. Tb Menopace ISO	

Multi Vitamin (To make diet more complete)

i. Becosule	
ii. Reconia	
iii. Cevit	Rs. 5-8 / capsule
iv. Cobadex	
v. Tb Fefol (Iron)	

Drug Prices – Then and Now

Way back in 1970 when Late Smt. Indira Gandhi was the prime minister of India, a committee was appointed to look into the drug scene including the patents act. The Hathi Committee recommended process patents instead of product patents leading to no legal hindrance in manufacturing of molecules by reverse engineering by pharma companies. Thus, for last 38 years drug prices were not high in India unlike foreign countries, any of which one ruled by product patents. Obviously the poor people of India couldn't have got a better deal. But, now India is in transition phase and the product patents regime and intellectual property rights are the order of the day. Most of the molecules are out of its ambit for now but same cannot be said for the future. The only solace is indigenous research and development, on fast track.

Chapter 13
Case History of Patients

Renu Dhall, (India)

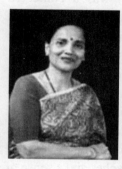

Renu Dhall, (India) 56, is a former school teacher. Since the age of 40, she has suffered extreme back pain. 'I couldn't stand, and I was in so much pain that I couldn't even sit down without great discomfort' she recalls. Mrs Dhall consulted several doctors, but none of them diagnosed her problem as osteoporosis. 'They told me back pain is common in women after multiple pregnancies, or it's related to your periods, or get your kidneys checked. The only common refrain I heard from the doctors was take some pain killers and learn to live with it.'

During the period that Mrs Dhall suffered without a diagnosis, her mother suffered multiple fractures and was confined to bed. Still, no one told Mrs Dhall about osteoporosis.

A few years ago Mrs Dhall read in the Hindustan Times about a bone densitometry camp, she got a bone densitometry test done and was diagnosed with osteoporosis and offered treatment. After spending years in agony, Mrs Dhall got what she terms 'a new lease on life'.

Since joining a local osteoporosis support group, she says 'My outlook on life is much better.' Mrs Dhall exercises regularly and has learned guidelines to reduce the risk of fracture. Mrs Dhall feels so much better in fact, that she was able to return to teaching. Although unable to work her usual hours, Mrs Dhall finds happiness in teaching shorter periods at a more leisurely pace.

Her message to others is simple – 'Do not put up with pain. Insist that your doctor test you for osteoporosis'.

Ram Gulam, (India)

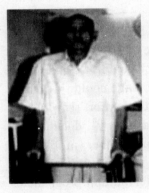

Ram Gulam, (India) was a contented man. He was a respected panch (head of the village council) in the Indian village of Larpur, in the District of Azamgarh, a hamlet of 5000 people in the state of Uttar Pradesh. He was also a well-to-do farmer, owning land and a small cattle ranch. Pictures of Ram Gulam show a tall, proud, good looking 58-year-old man, with big moustaches and a sense of self-confidence.

One sunny morning Ram Gulam shared tea session with fellow villagers and discussed an important judgement he was going to make later in the day at the village council meeting. Promised to objectively review both sides of the case, involving a land dispute, and excused himself to prepare for the meeting.

While in the bath Ram Gulam slipped and fell. 'The fall was trivial,' he recalls, 'but the pain was excruciating.' He could not stand and his family took him to the district hospital, at Azamgarh, 40 kms away from his village. After an X-ray, the doctor on duty diagnosed a fracture to the neck of the femur and told him that he would need surgery.

Not convinced that such a small fall could cause a fracture needing surgery, he was brought by his relatives to Delhi, some 400 kms away. There, Dr Sushil Sharma, an orthopaedic surgeon closely associated with the Arthritis Foundation of India, explained that Ram Gulam had broken the head of his femur, commonly called a hip fracture, because of weak bones. Ram Gulam was operated upon and then began a long and painful rehabilitation, during which his job as community affairs judge in the local council was provisionally taken over by another person.

Only after four months he could resume light exercises and a normal life, Ram Gulam recalls, 'but I remained skeptical of my doctor's diagnosis that I had osteoporosis – I was convinced that weak bones was a disease of women, not men,' he says. A few months later while on one of his evening walks, Ram Gulam made a quick movement to dodge a stray dog. He slipped, fell, and fractured his other hip. Again he saw the surgeon, and again he had a hip replacement surgery. But this time his rehabilitation was much more difficult. He was bedridden. Once again he lost his panchayat decision-making position at the village community court. His esteem was gone and he had become isolated.

Today Ram Gulam is an ill and depressed man. He can walk with the help of a walker, but at the age of 65 he looks like 90. He has started osteoporosis treatment, but after his two hip fractures the weak bones have already taken their toll.

After his second hip surgery he went for a BMD check. His T-score was -4.9, and his spine showed evidence of vertebral collapse. He has lost 4 cm in height in the past seven years, and he is in constant pain. As he gets around the hospital corridors with his walker, Ram Gulam is totally heart broken – he has now been told that his job as the village council head has been permanently given to another man. Things could have been better had he taken care of osteoporosis at the right time.

Dan Martell, USA

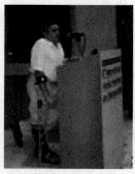

What happens to a man who, at the age of 33, realizes that his life has been irreversibly turned upside down? Dan experienced chronic foot pain in 1988. None of the specialists he consulted could accurately diagnosis his osteoporosis – they suggested his problem may be due to arthritis or possibly psychosomatic illness.

The following year he fractured a vertebra, and a bone density test revealed that he had lost 70 percent of his bone mass. Dan has had more operations than he can remember; including seven surgeries on his hips to implant various plates and screws. Steel rods have been inserted in both his femurs.

Dan, now 55, has fractured every vertebra in his back and fractures his ribs almost monthly. 'My ribs or vertebra can fracture from simply coughing or sneezing' he says. In spite of his continuing fractures, Dan feels that 'my fracture rate would be even higher without the medication that I've been prescribed'.

He has lost 23 cm in height, and is mostly confined to a wheelchair. 'I can no longer play with my son, ride a bike with my daughter or walk on the beach with my wife,' he explains. He was forced to resign his job as maintenance supervisor for a major beverage production plant. 'Osteoporosis is not just a disease of the elderly,' he says. 'It can be very debilitating and extremely painful'. Dan recommends that people should talk to their physicians about the risks of osteoporosis and insist on a bone density test when it is indicated. In spite of the fact that Dan and his mother had osteoporosis, both of his sisters had to insist that their physicians give them a bone density test. 'Both were found to have low bone density,' he notes, 'and are taking medication so they don't wind up like me'.

Salima Ladak-Kachra, Canada

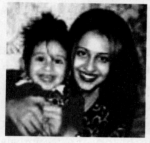

At the age of 25, I sustained four compression fractures in my spine when I slipped and fell on a ceramic floor. When I hit the floor, I felt unbearable pain course down my back. I almost urinated in my pants, the pain was so excruciating. I couldn't move my body and for a moment, I thought I was paralysed. I couldn't stop crying. I knew something terrible had happened.

The next thing I knew, I was in the emergency department. No one could understand why I was in so much pain and why I couldn't get up. An x-ray showed that I had crushed my vertebrae. The emergency physician was shocked to see what appeared on the X-ray. He said the damage to my back looked as though someone had hammered it with a baseball bat.

Most people who fall and land on their backs usually have little discomfort or minor soft tissue injury. However, I was an exception to that rule. I experienced excruciating pain and was not able to walk, shower, eat or dress myself without assistance. I truly felt physically handicapped. I discovered that I had lost one inch in height and my waist increased from 18 to 22 inches. I had trouble performing daily tasks such as cooking, doing the laundry and cleaning. I felt as though as I was eighty years old, fragile and weak.

I kept asking myself, Why is this happening to me? I was so young and had my entire life ahead of me. I was newly married and was planning on having children in the near future. With the constant pain in my entire back, I began to suffer both physically and emotionally and went through a period of depression. This depression also put a strain on my marriage as I had trouble communicating and being intimate due to the unbearable pain. The pain medications made me feel sleepy and lethargic, but thank goodness they worked.

Prior to my fractures, I had seen a few physicians for back pain, but then I was told that I was guilty of nothing more than improper body mechanics! The apparent risk factors I had for osteoporosis were ignored, probably due to my young age. After all, osteoporosis had always been associated with hunched-over elderly women. I have a very strong family history of osteoporosis on both sides of my family. I also have a petite body frame and I am of Asian descent. I had low calcium intake throughout my adolescent years, because I had difficulty tolerating dairy products and barely focused on being physically active.

In addition, my menstrual cycle was irregular virtually from its onset. At age 20, after suffering a severe weight loss (a pixie-like 87 pounds), nausea and headaches, my new family physician ordered comprehensive blood and diagnostic tests. These revealed that I had hyperprolactinemia. This condition, along with the other aforementioned factors were preventing me from attaining my peak bone mass and as a result, my bones were thin.

It was only the very painful experience of four vertebral fractures that forced an investigation of my bone health. A bone density examination revealed severe osteopenia in both my spine and femur regions, requiring immediate measures to be taken. To this day, I still do not have back pain and neither my body feels nor looks the same as it once did. I still have trouble cleaning the house, making the bed or being in one position for a prolonged period of time. I am now committed to preventing anyone from enduring the same experience that I underwent.

It is vital for one to have optimal Calcium intake, to practise regular weight-bearing exercise, restrain from excess caffeine or alcohol consumption and to not smoke. These are only a few of the risk factors for osteoporosis. Osteoporosis is a multi-factorial disease that can happen to anyone regardless of gender or ethnic background or age.

If there was more focus on the awareness and knowledge of different osteoporosis risk factors, achieving peak bone mass and diagnosis of low bone mass in young women, perhaps I would not have fractured my bones. My experience has provided me with the motivation to be an advocate for women's health education. I believe all women, regardless of age or ethnic background, deserve access to health education and to be informed of the risk factors and preventive measures for osteoporosis. If I make a difference in even one woman's life, it is a reward that I will hold to be truly priceless.

Chapter 14
Physiotherapy Gadgets

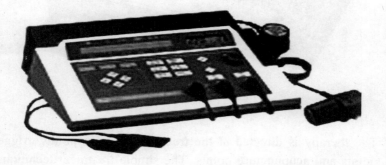

Combination Unit for Ultrasound, Electro and Combination Therapy

- Continuous and pulsed ultrasound therapy
- 1 and 3 MHz
- Connection for two treatment heads simultaneously
- Contact control-Automatic power switch-off and treatment time interruption in case of insufficeint contact. The visual indicator of the treatment head swithes on
- Three current types for electrotherapy
- Combination of ultrasound with either one of the three current types.
- Use – Pain relief, nerve stimulation, lymphatic drainage and to alleviate symptoms due to nerve compression etc.

Infra-Red Laser therapy

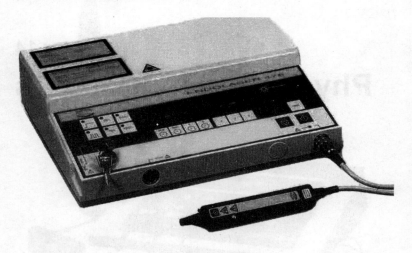

The therapy is directed at the treatment of pain points, trigger points and acupuncture points. The simple treatment technique, the relatively short treatment times and good clinical results obtained offer clear advantages.

- Continuous and pulsed laser therapy
- Easy adjustment of the dosage
- Automatic calculation of the treatment time
- 2 different laser probes with target indication
- Conveniently arranged control panel
- Portable because of battery supply
- Use – Beneficial in acute traumatic conditions and pain healing

Universal traction unit for lumbar and cervical traction

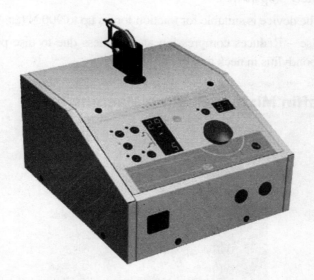

Continuous and intermittent traction

The traction force of this device can be set to continuous or intermittent. A special control must be pressed for traction forces above 200 N (ca. 20 kg). This safety system prevents accidental unacceptable high traction forces during, for instance, cervical traction.

Safety

The control panel shows various parameters which can be selected with fingertips controls like traction force, base force, base hold time and treatment time. The traction force is electronically measured and constantly monitored. A microcomputer compares the actual readings with the set values and immediately eliminates any differences. Patient movement is recorded and does not influence the traction force. The patient can gradually reduce the traction power to the minimum value (15 N) by simply pressing the safety stop switch.

The device is suitable for traction forces up to 900 N (ca. 90 kg).

Use – Reduces compression and stiffness due to disc prolapse and spondylitis in neck and back.

Paraffin Mixture Beating Machine

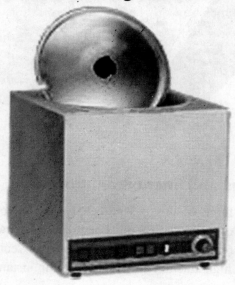

The device is a beating unit for **paraffin mixtures**. The compact design as table model makes the unit suitable to be used in any kind of practice. It is possible to process paraligno as well as Parafango Battaglia in the heater. Because of the direct heating system, this device is highly suitable for sterilising paraffin wax (at 135C). Sterilising is only possible when Parafango Battaglia is used (paraligno cannot stand these high temperatures). It is glass wool insulated and is supplied as standard with a splash cover with cold grip.

Paraligno

Paraligno is composed out of **paraffin mixed with birch sawdust**. It can be used for any packing size. Paraligno has long term of heat development.

Parafango Battaglia

Parafango is composed out of paraffin mixed with fango (mud). It can be used for any packing size. Parafango has a long term of heat development. Frequently heating for sterilisation (130 140 C) does not harm the Parafango.

Paraffin Bath

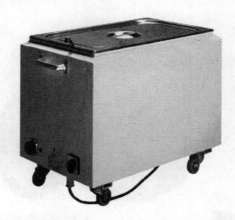

The paraffin bath operates on the 'au bain-marie' principle; the paraffin is heated directly by the heat transferred from a heat transfer liquid.

The advantages are:
- Quicker heating
- More even heat distribution
- Practically no temperature fluctuations in the paraffin

As heat-transfer liquid you can use water or a special thermal-oil. For sterilisation of pure paraffin the use of a special thermal oil is necessary (or else the required temperature cannot be reached). The bath is mobile and contains a stainless steel inner tank with splash cover. The bath is equipped with an electric heating element with thermostatic temperature control (30-90° C) and an overheating safety mechanism.

The wide sizes of the bath makes it suitable for so called dipping treatments. It is possible to heat Paraligno, Parafango and pure paraffin in this bath.

Paraffin

Pure form paraffin with a melting point of 48°-52°C.

Packheater

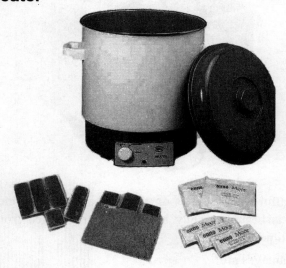

The Packheater is used for heating of packs. The enamelled heater is standard delivered including base grid. The water temperature is accurately maintained by a thermostat at a pre-selected, constant value (50-95°C).

Use – Provides superficial heating and reduces pain and inflammation.

Synthetic heat pack

Synthetic pack filled with 'moor' because of the special filling gives off heat extremely slowly. The pack can also be heated in a Microwave.

Hot/Cold pack

Synthetic pack filled with gel. The pack can also be heated in a Microwave.

Microwave Therapy Unit (Short Wave Diathermy)

This device is a unit for microwave therapy. This unit for heat therapy offers a choice from continuous or pulsed output.

Continuous or pulsed output

A choice can be made from a continuous output of maximum 250 watt or pulsed output with a maximum of 1500 watt which makes it possible to heat up deeper lying tissues with a low dosage.

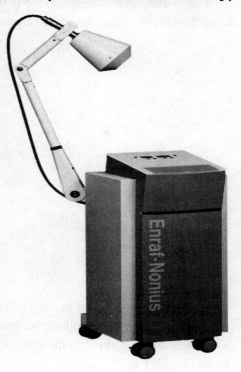

Effortless transition between continuous and pulsed therapy

During the course of treatment you can easily switch from continuous to pulsed output. In the meantime the electronic system keeps the effective dosage constant.

Simple operation and clear reproduction

Dosage and treatment time are digitally displayed on screen. They are easy to set with the push buttons. The different radiators can easily be attached to the adjustable arm by means of a practical quick coupling. The treatment starts as soon as the power is set. The unit automatically turns off and gives an audible signal when the treatment time ends.

Use – The deep heating device is used for reducing pain and inflammation and can cover large areas also.

Chapter 15
Recipes

Indian Dish Made from Mixed Grains and Rice

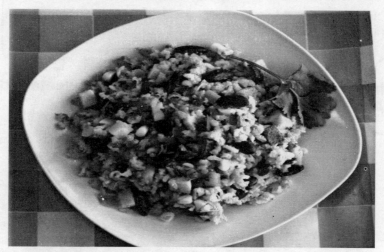

Ingredients

Pounded pearl millet	-	250 gm
Pounded Finger millet	-	50 gm
Green bean	-	50 gm
Rice	-	50 gm
Salt	-	According to taste
Cumin seeds	-	1tsp
Turmeric powder	-	1tsp

Water	-	3 glasses
Oil	-	1 tbsp

Method of Preparation

i. Soak grains and pulses for an hour.
ii. Put them in a pressure cooker and cook for 15 minutes.
iii. Heat oil, add cumin seeds and pour this seasoning on the cooked grains and pulses.
iv. Garnish with green chilly and lemon, serve hot.

Serves—4

Nutritive value per serving

Energy	-	350 kcal
Protein	-	12.1 gm
Calcium	-	86 mg

Indian Dish with Cottage cheese and Sweetened Ash Gourd

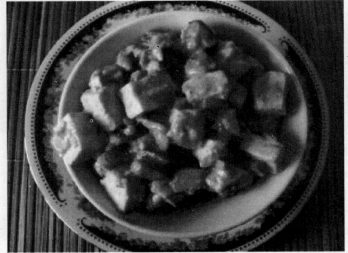

Ingredients

Cottage cheese	-	250 gm, grated
Ash gourd and sugar preparation	-	200 gm, grated

Coconut powder	-	100 gm
Almonds	-	10 gm

Method of Preparation

i. Keep aside 50 gm coconut powder.
ii. Add remaining coconut powder to grated Cottage cheese and ash gourd and mix well.
iii. Roll this mixture into small balls with buttered hands.
iv. Roll in coconut powder and garnish with almonds.

Serves–10

Nutritive value per serving (2ps)

Energy	-	224.5 kcal
Protein	-	5.11 gm
Calcium	-	204 mg

Dessert Made from Indian Cottage Cheese and Cream

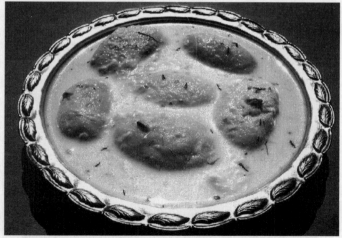

Ingredients

Orange pulp	-	200 gm
Indian cottage cheese	-	250 gm

Buffalo's milk	-	2 ltr
Sugar	-	150 gm

Method of Preparation

i. Mix half of orange pulp with Indian cottage cheese. Make small balls of this mixture.
ii. Put these balls in the boiling sugar syrup and cook for 15 minutes. Sweetened balls are ready.
iii. Boil buffalo's milk. When reduced to half, add sugar in it.
iv. Cool this and add other half of orange pulp.
v. Finally, add sliced sweetened balls in this condensed milk and serve chilled.

Serves–5

Nutritive value per serving (2ps)

Energy	-	700 kcal
Protein	-	27 gm
Calcium	-	954.4 mg

Egg Custard

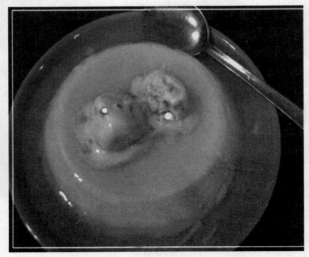

Ingredients

Milk	-	200 ml
Egg	-	1
Sugar	-	2 tsp
Vanilla essence	-	3-4 drops
Custard powder	-	1 tsp

Method of Preparation

i. Simmer milk in a wok. Add custard powder.
ii. Beat egg and sugar in a pan.
iii. Pour milk gradually over the egg mixture.
iv. Keep the pan over fire. Stir constantly until the custard start coating on the spoon and add vanilla essence.
v. Cool and keep it in the refrigerator. Serve chilled.

Serves–2

Nutritive value per serving

Energy	-	196 kcal
Protein	-	7.6 mg
Calcium	-	225 mg

Fish Pizza

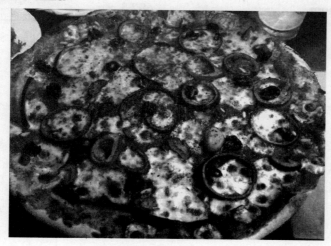

Ingredients

Pizza base	-	1
Chopped soya leaves	-	50 gm
Boiled fish	-	200 gm
Cucumber (sliced)	-	1
Cheese (grated)	-	50 gm
Tomato sauce	-	2 tbsp
Oil	-	1 tsp

Method of Preparation

i. Toss pizza base with oil.
ii. Spread tomato sauce over it and put soya leaves.
iii. Now put fish slices and cucumber slices on it.
iv. Sprinkle cheese and grill for 15 minutes.

Serves–2

Nutritive value per serving

Energy	-	149.8 kcal
Protein	-	20 gm
Calcium	-	697.3 mg

Roasted Chick Pea Shake

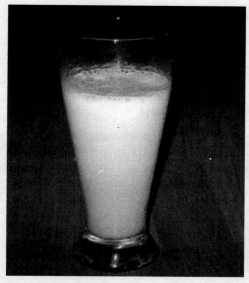

Ingredients

Roasted chick pea	-	100 gm
Milk	-	400 ml
Sugar	-	25 gm
Cardamom powder	-	½ tsp
Ice		

Method of Preparation

i. Remove seed coat and make a fine powder of roasted chick pea in mixture.
ii. Mix chick pea powder, cardamom powder, sugar and milk in a blender.
iii. Serve chilled.

Serves–2	
Nutritive value per serving	
Energy	- 468.5 kcal
Protein	- 19.85 gm
Calcium	- 450 mg

Spinach tomato Soup

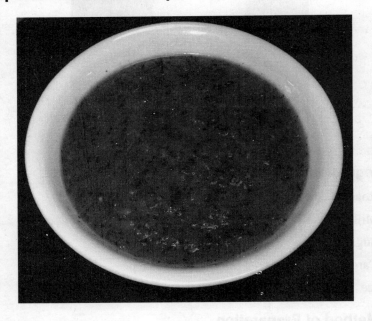

Ingredients

Tomatoes	– 3-4 finely sliced
Lamb's quarters	– 50 gm
Spinach	– 1 bunch
Onion	– ½ large, finely sliced
Water	– 2-3 cups

Garlic	–	6-7 cloves
Ginger	–	½ inch piece, finely sliced
Salt and pepper	–	according to taste
Refined flour	–	1 tbsp
Cream	–	½ tsp for garnishing

Method of Preparation

i. Pressure cook all the ingredients for 10-15 minutes.
ii. Mix it with a blender.
iii. Finely strain through a stainless steel/mesh strainer.
iv. Again heat and pour into individual soup bowls.
v. Garnish with cream.
vi. Serve hot.

Calcium content - 190 mg

Fenugreek Mushroom Soup

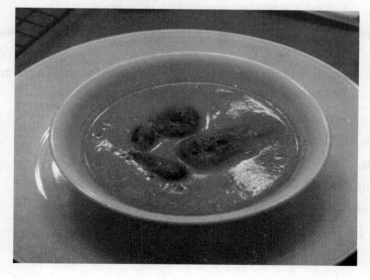

Ingredients

Mushrooms	–	½ packet, finely sliced
Onions	–	½ large, finely sliced
Fenugreek leaves	–	few leaves finely sliced
Water	–	½ cup
White flour	–	1 tbsp
Vegetable oil	–	1 tbsp
Soya Sauce	–	½ tbsp
White button mushrooms	–	½ packet, finely sliced
Salt and pepper	–	according to taste
Cream	–	for garnishing
Low fat milk	–	½ cup

Method of Preparation

i. Semi-heat the olive oil and saute the onions.
ii. Add the mushrooms and slightly saute them.
iii. Add the flour and quickly mix with the onions and mushrooms on low heat.
iv. Slowly add the heated milk water mixture, so that lumps are not formed. Boil it and add the salt and pepper.
v. Turn off the heat.
vi. Add coriander leaves.
vii. At last, add the soya sauce and blend into the soup.
viii. Garnish with cream and serve hot.

Calcium content – 55mg

Sprouts Salad

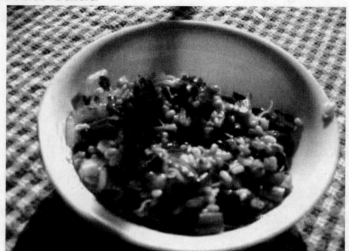

Ingredients

Red chillies	–	2-4 grounded
Ginger	–	1 inch piece, sliced finely
Cloves	–	5 cloves, sliced finely
Soya chunks	–	100 gm, mashed
Salt	–	½ tsp
Vegetable oil	–	1½ tbsp
Soya bean sprouts	–	500 gm
Garlic	–	2 piece, finely sliced

Method of Preparation

i. Semi-heat the oil in a non-stick wok and fry the mashed soya chunks with salt, until it is golden brown. Remove it from heat.

ii. Put the chilli and ginger paste in the left over oil.

iii. Add the bean sprouts and stir-fry for about 1 minute.

Calcium content - 350 mg

Mixed Veg Salad

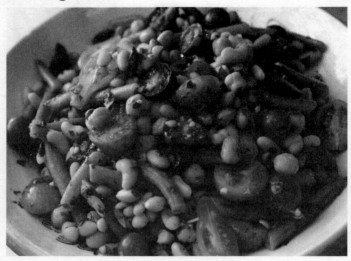

Ingredients

Kidney beans	– 1 cup, soaked overnight, boiled and drained
Cow pea	– 1 cup, boiled
Black gram	– 1 cup
Vegetable oil	– 1 tbsp
Vinegar	– 1 tbsp
Amla juice	– 1tsp
Sugar	– 2 tbsp
Salt/Pepper	– according to taste

Method of Preparation

i. Mix all three beans.
ii. Add all ingredients.
iii. Bake for 25-30 min.
iv. Serve while hot.

Calcium content - 160 mg

Soya Rice

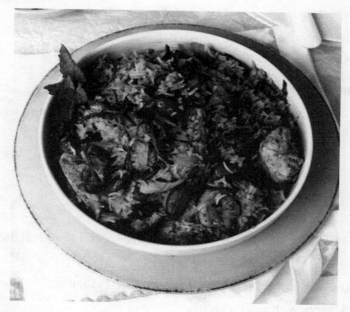

Ingredients

Soya chunks	– 350 gm, soaked in lukewarm water and drained
Brown rice	– 2 cups, washed and drained
Turmeric powder	– 1/2 tsp
Onions	– 6 thinly sliced length wise
Garlic	– 10-12 cloves, crushed
Ginger	– 2 inch piece, crushed
Bay leaves	– 2
Cinnamon	– 5-6 sticks
Cardamom	– 4-5
Cloves	– ½ tsp

Vegetable oil	– 2 tbsp
Cardamom	– 4-5
Salt	– according to taste
Cottage cheese	– 50 gm

Method of Preparation

i. Heat oil in pan, add the cloves, cinnamon, cardamon and tej patta.

ii. As they splutter add the onions and fry them till they get slightly brown.

iii. Add the ginger garlic paste and fry for 2-3 minutes.

iv. Add the rice and fry for a minute or two.

v. Add the soya chunks, salt and move around for 30 seconds.

vi. Add cottage cheese.

vii. Cook on very low heat for about 15-20 minutes.

viii. Serve with green chutney.

Calcium content - 260 mg

Vegetable Medley

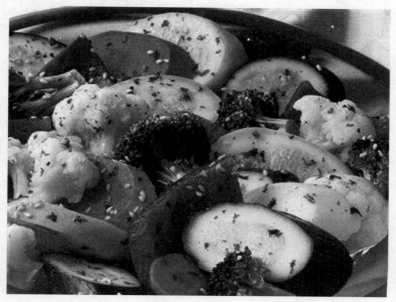

Ingredients

Garlic	—	4-5 cloves, crushed
Green chilli	—	2, finely sliced
Fenugreek leaves	—	8 stalks, sliced
Vegetable oil	—	1½ tsp
Butter milk	—	1 cup
Salt	—	according to taste

Method of Preparation

i. Mix all the ingredients in a bowl.
ii Place at the centre of a plateful of bread cut into pieces.
iii. Serve.

Calcium content - 90 mg

Cottage Cheese and Corn

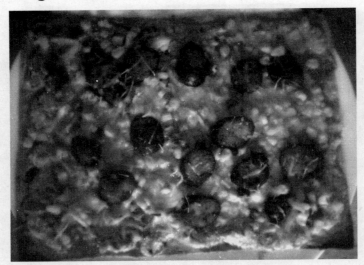

Ingredients

Fresh cottage cheese	–	250 gm
Steamed corns	–	175 gm
Cumin seeds	–	½ tsp
Vegetable oil	–	1 tsp
White mustard seeds	–	½ tsp

Method of Preparation

i. Semi-heat the oil, in a non-stick wok.

ii. Add the cumin seeds and mustard seeds.

iii. When they begin to splutter, add the crushed cottage cheese.

iv. Add the corn and the salt.

v. Cook lightly for 5-7 minutes.

vi. Serve.

Calcium content - 500mg

Hearty Vegetable Medley

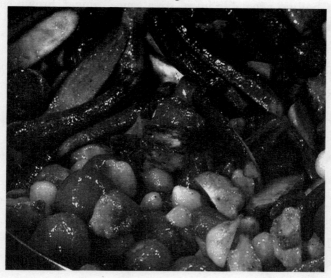

Ingredients

Brown rice	–	2 cups
Broccoli	–	2 whole
Lotus stem	–	100gm
Vegetable juice	–	½ cup
Tomato sauce	–	2 tbsp
Regular tofu	–	500 gm
Fresh ginger	–	1 inch piece, sliced
Brown sugar	–	2 tbsp
Chilli flakes	–	½ tbsp
Foil		

Method of Preparation
i. Steam rice.

ii. In a large, shallow pan, set a rack over approximatley 1 inch of boiling vegetable juice, soya sauce, ginger, brown sugar and chilli flakes.
iii. Drain tofu and cut into pieces.
iv. Turn the tofu into the broth.
v. Remove and gently place the tofu on to the rack.
vi. Covering the pan with a foil and steam it for 10 minutes.
vii. Remove the rack of tofu.
viii. Add water to the broth to make it 1 inch deep and add the broccoli.
ix. Cook for about 4 minutes, until it is tender and can be pierced comfortably.
x. Take out broccoli.
xi. Serve rice in the bowls with the broth, broccoli, tofu and boiled lotus stem.
xii. Add tomato sauce for taste, if required.
xiii. Serve

Calcium content - 300 mg

Prawn Curry

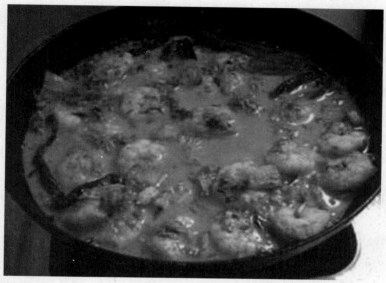

Ingredients

Prawns	–	250gm, cleaned
Sardines	–	250gm
Coconut milk	–	1.5 cups
Onions	–	2, finely sliced
Turmeric	–	½ tsp
Dry red chillies	–	4, grounded
Ginger juice	–	1tbsp
Vegetable oil	–	1 ½ tbsp
Bay leaf	–	1 large
Cloves	–	5-6
Cinnamon	–	2-3 inch-sized pieces
Cardamon	–	2-3

Seasonings (powder of clove – cardamom and cinnamon)	½ tsp
Salt	– according to taste
Sugar	– a pinch

Method of Preparation

i. Semi-heat the oil in a non-stick pan and add the bay leaves, cardamom, cinnamon and cloves.
ii. When they start spluttering, add the sliced onions and fry till they are golden brown.
iii. Add the turmeric and chilli paste and cook for 20-30 seconds.
iv. Add the ginger juice and cook for 30 seconds.
v. Add the prawns and sardines, cook and mix it well.
vi. Add salt and sugar.
vii. Pour the coconut milk and bring to a boil.
viii. Quickly turn off the heat, do not overcook.
ix. Add garam masala.
x. Serve with steamed rice.

Calcium content – 600 mg

Heart Healthy Steamed Fish

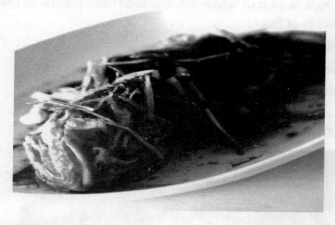

Ingredients

Coconut	–	½ scrapped
Shell fish	–	½ kg, washed
Mint leaves	–	half bunch
Garlic	–	1 whole pod
Ginger	–	1-2 inch piece
Lemon juice	–	1
Olive oil	–	1½ tsp
Salt	–	according to taste
Banana leaves foil		

Method of Preparation

i. Prepare a chutney with all the ingredients other than the fish, oil and banana leaves foil.
ii. Liberally oil the insides of the banana leaves.

iii. Wrap fish into banana leaves and make a neat parcel of it, a single in case of whole fish and individual parcels in case of pieces of fish.
iv. Steam for 20 minutes.
v. Serve.

Calcium content - 550mg

Nutritious Combi-Dombi Salad

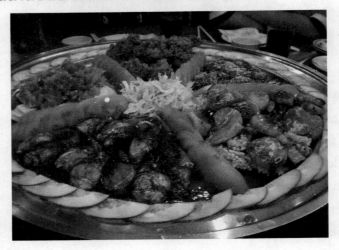

Ingredients

Cottage cheese	–	100 gm
Onions	–	2, medium chopped
Cumin seeds	–	1 tsp roasted
Garlic	–	4 flakes, sliced finely
Green chillies	–	2 sliced finely
Turmeric powder	–	½ tsp
Black pepper powder	–	1 tsp
Tomatoes	–	2 medium, chopped

Curry leaves	–	a bunch, chopped
Mayonnaise	–	1tsp
Salt/Pepper	–	according to taste
Nuts	–	50 gm
Vegetable oil	–	1tsp

Method of Preparation

i. Semi-heat the oil in a non-stick pan and add the cumin seeds.
ii. When they splutter, add the curry leaves, green chillies and the garlic.
iii. Stir-fry for 15-30 sec.
iv. Add the chopped onions and saute for a few minutes.
v. Add the chopped tomatoes, turmeric powder, salt and pepper.
vi. Cook this mixture till the oil begins to float on top.
vii. Add the black pepper.
viii. Add the cottage cheese and mix well.
ix. Cover for a few minutes.
x. Garnish with nuts.
xi. Serve.

Calcium content - 920 mg

Lotus Root Salad

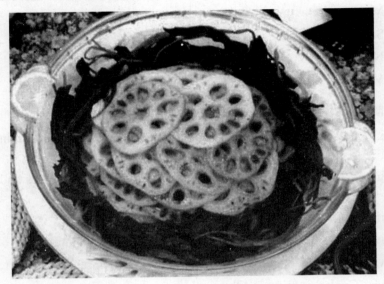

Ingrdients

Lotus root	– 2 stalks, steamed for 3 minutes and cut into inch-sized strips
Cucumber	– ½ peeled and cut finely
Fresh spinach leaves	– About 10-12, finely chopped
Lemon juice	– 1 lemon
Red chillies	– 2-3, finely chopped
Soya sauce	– 2 tbsp
Garlic	– 2 cloves, crushed
Sugar	- 1 tbsp

Method of Preparation

i. Make a dressing of lemon juice, chillies, fish sauce, garlic and sugar, set aside.

ii. Mix the cucumber, lotus stem and fresh spinach leaves, making sure that all the water has been drained.
iii. Add the dressing and chill in the refrigerator for 20 minutes before serving.

Calcium content - 340 mg

Garlicky Crabs Delight

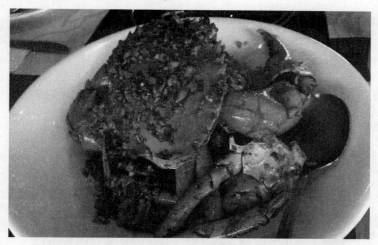

Ingredients

Crabs	—	2 large; 6 small, finely cut into pieces.
Garlic	—	2 pods, roughly crushed
Pepper	—	1 tsp
Vegtable oil	—	3 tsp
Salt	—	according to taste

Method of Preparation

i. In a large bowl, boil water in it.
ii. Throw in the crabs and blanch for 2-3 minutes; drain.

iii. Semi heat the oil in a non-stick wok, throw in the crushed garlic. Fry until light golden brown.
iv. Add the crabs and toss in the garlic for 2 minutes.
v. Add the salt and pepper.
vi. Serve hot.

Calcium content - 1300 mg

Low Calorie Spinach Yoghurt

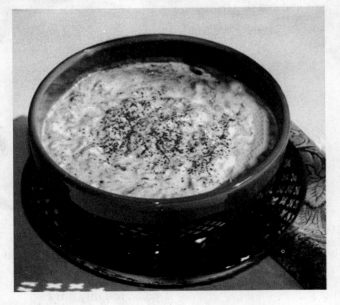

Ingredients

Thick yoghurt	– 200 gm
Spinach	– 1 bunch, chopped fine length wise and blanched for a minute in hot water and drained
Cumin powder	– ½ tsp
Salt	– according to taste

Rock salt	– ½ tsp
Asafoetida	– 1 pinch

Method of Preparation

i. Mix all the ingredients in a bowl.
ii. Transfer to a serving bowl.
iii. Garnish it with cumin powder.
iv. Seasoning with asafoetida and ½ tsp of oil.

Calcium content -220 mg

Banana Smoothie

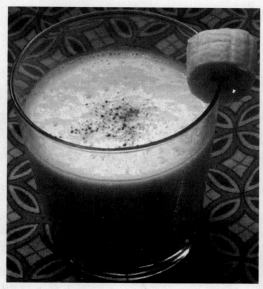

Ingredients

Milk	– ½ kg
Ripe banana	– 1
Sugar/Splenda	– 1 tsp

Butterscotch essence	–	1 drop
Ice	–	½ cup
Almonds	–	4
Cashewnuts	–	4

Method of Preparation

i. Mix all the ingredients in a blender for 3 minutes till it is thick and frothy.
ii. Pour it in the glass.
iii. Serve chilled.
iv. Garnish with nuts.

Calcium content - 184 mg

Spinach Salad

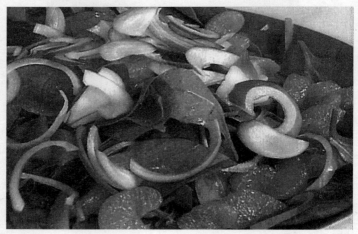

Ingredients

Spinach leaves	–	1 cup, torn
Mandarin oranges	–	¼ cup
Balsamic vinegar	–	2 tbsp

Method of Preparation
i. Mix ingredients together.
ii. Serve with lunch and dinner.

Cacium Content – 180mg

Stir Fry Chicken and Broccoli

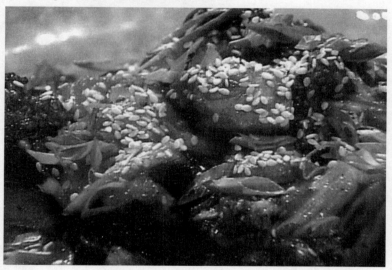

Ingredients

Extra virgin olive oil	– 2 tbsp
Free range organic chicken breasts	– 2, cut into thin strips
Garlic	– 2, crushed
Cloves	– 2, crushed
Fresh root ginger	– 1 inch piece, grated
Broccoli	– 1, cut into small florets
Spring onions	– 6, finely sliced

Mushrooms	– ½ cup, halved
Bean sprouts	– 3 ounces
Oyster sauce	– 3 tbsp
Soy sauce	– 1 tbsp
Chicken stock	– 4 ounces
Lemon Juice	– ½ lemon

Method of Preparation

i. Heat 1 tablespoon of olive oil in a large pan or wok and add the chicken strips.

ii. Fry for approximately 5 minutes turning continuously and until cooked through.

iii. Remove from pan onto plate and set aside.

iv. Heat the remaining 1 tablespoon of oil in the same pan.

v. Add the ginger and garlic.

vi. Cook on low heat for approximately 1 minute taking care not to burn the garlic. Add the broccoli, onions and mushrooms and cook for a further 5 minutes.

vii. Return the chicken to the pan and add the sprouts, soy and oyster sauce, stock and lemon juice. Cook for a further 1 to 2 minutes. Toss well and serve.

viii. Sprinkle with cashew nuts if desired.

Cacium content – 500mg

Wheat Soya Mix

Ingredients
Whole wheat	– 80 gm
Whole soyabean	– 20 gm

Method of Preparation
i. Clean whole wheat and soyabean separately.
ii. Roast wheat and soyabean in hot sand.
iii. Grind these separately and mix together.
iv. Store the prepared instant food in an air tight container.

Calcium Content-160mg

Broken Wheat Mix

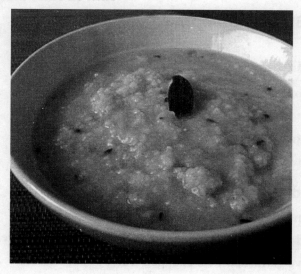

Ingredients
Broken wheat	– 40 gm
Green gram	– 20 gm

Groundnut	–	10 gm
Sugar	–	30 gm
Oil	–	2 tbsp

Method of Preparation

i. Roast broken wheat, green gram and groundnuts separately.
ii. Heat oil in a wok and add roasted broken wheat and green gram.
iii. When it turns brown, add water to it.
iv. Then add sugar and wait till water has evaporated.
v. Sprinkle with cardamon powder.
vi. Serve hot with groundnuts.

Calcium content-34mg

Tofu Banana Smoothie

Ingredients

Silken tofu	–	300 gm
Banana	–	1, ripe
Orange juice	–	½ cup
Sugar or honey	–	1 tbsp

Method of Preparation

i. Blend all the ingredients in a mixer until smooth.
ii. Add some crushed ice and blend for a 30 second cycle.
iii. Serve garnished with chopped fruit of your choice.

Calcium content-200mg

Strawberry Raisin Yoghurt Smoothie

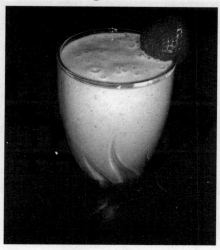

Ingredients

Fresh or frozen strawberries	–	1 cup
Cashew nut powder	–	1 tbsp, (cashew nuts lightly toasted and powdered)
Raisins	–	2 tbsp
Yoghurt (curd)	–	1 cup, chilled
Sugar or honey	–	1 tsp

Method of Preparation

i. Blend all the ingredients till smooth and creamy.
ii. Serve garnished with chopped strawberries or nuts of your choice.

Calcium content- 121mg

Cheesy Mushroom Omelette

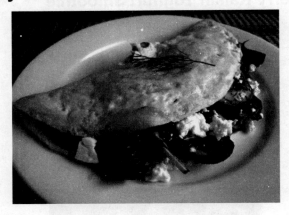

Serves - 1

Ingredients

Egg	–	2
Water	–	2 tbsp
Low fat cheese	–	50 gm
Tomatoes	–	150 gm
Finely chopped parsley	–	¼ cup
Button mushrooms	–	200 gm
Water	–	¼ cup extra
Pepper	–	according to taste
Chopped parsley	–	for garnishing

Method of Preparation

i. Wrisk eggs and water in a bowl until just combined. In a separate bowl, mix cheese, tomatoes and 2 tablespoons of parsley.

ii. Pour half the egg mixture into a non-stick frying pan to just cover the base. Cook over medium heat until eggs are almost set. Place half the cheese mixture over the omelette and fold in half. Slide onto a serving dish, deep warm and repeat with remaining mixture to make another omelette.

iii. Heat non-stick frying pan and add mushrooms and water and saute until cooked through. Use seasoning for better taste and stir in remaining parsley.

iv. Serve mushrooms on the cheesy omelette sprinkled with chopped parsley.

Calcium content - 286 mg

Spinach in Bengal Gram Pulse

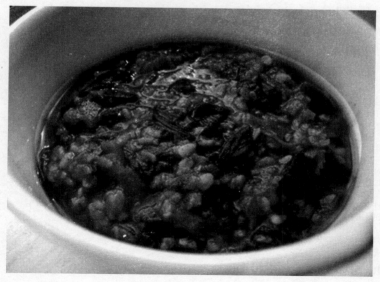

Ingredients

Bengal gram   —   80 gm

Spinach (chopped)	–	500 gm
Vegetable oil	–	2 tbsp
Coriander powder	–	1 tbsp
Red chilly powder	–	1 tbsp
Salt	–	1½ tbsp
Cumin seeds	–	1 tbsp
Asafoetida	–	½ tbsp
Ginger and green chilly paste	–	1 tbsp

Note: You can replace spinach with amaranth leaves.

Method of Preparation

i. Wash the bengal gram and chopped spinach well, separately.
ii. Boil bengal gram along with coriander powder, red chilly powder and salt.
iii. Add the chopped spinach to the bengal gram and cook it for another 5 minutes.
iv. Put ghee in a pan.
v. Let it heat and add cumin seeds, asafoetida, ginger and green chilly powder.
vi. Add the boiled gram and spinach mixture to it.
vii. Serve it with chapatti or rice.

Calcium content - 200 mg

Steamed and Sauted Colocasia Leaves

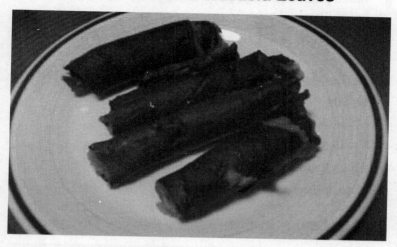

Serves - 2

Ingredients

Colocasia leaves	–	8
Oil	–	1½ tbsp
Seasoning	–	cumin and mustard seeds
Gramflour	–	200 gm
Ginger	–	25 gm
Garlic	–	10 cloves
Red chilli powder	–	5 gm
Salt and pepper	–	according to taste

Method of Preparation

i. Clean the leaves.

ii. Make a thick paste of gram flour, crushed ginger, garlic and red chilli powder.
iii. Put one leaf facing down and spread the gram flour paste on it.
iv. Make a layer of all the 8 leaves with the paste in between, ending with the gram flour paste.
v. Roll the leaves to make a 2 inch diameter toll.
vi. Steam it for about 10 minutes.
vii. Saute them with oil and seasonings.

Calcium content - 850 mg

Creamy Fruit Salad

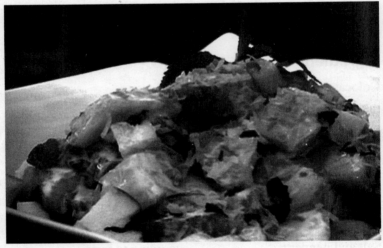

Serves - 10

Ingredients

Milk	–	2 kg
Fresh Cream	–	½ kg

Sugar	–	200 gm
Custard powder	–	4 tbsp
Apple	–	4 (pared and cut into small pieces)
Grapes	–	200 gm
Pomegranate	–	1 medium
Cashew nuts	–	50 gm
Vanilla essence	–	6 drops

Method of Preparation

i. Boil the milk and keep one half of a cup of milk and let it cool. Add sugar to the boiling milk.

ii. Add custard powder to the one half cup of cooled milk and mix it well to avoid knots and put it into the sugar and milk boiling mixture till it thickens.

iii. Let it cool in the refrigerator for a couple of hours.

iv. Once it is cooled, churn it with a hand mixer.

v. Churn the fresh cream mixed with a tablespoon full of powdered sugar with a hand mixer and place it on ice. Once the cream thickens stop churning. (excess churning will separate the cream out).

vi. Now put the thickened milk and cream together and churn it with a hand mixer.

vii. Add all the cut fruits and nuts. Mix it well with a spoon and add the vanilla essence and put it in the refrigerator to chill.

viii. Serve chilled.

Calcium content - 270 mg

Milk and Rice Pudding

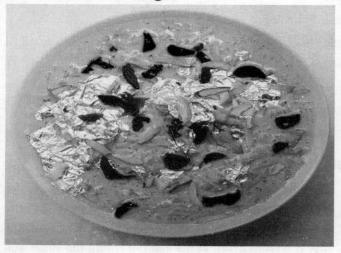

Serves - 4

Ingredients

Milk	–	1 kg
Rice (uncooked)	–	50 gms
Sugar	–	100 gms
Soaked and cut almonds and pistachio	–	1 tbsp
Cardamom powder	–	1 tbsp
Saffron leaves	–	5

Method of Preparation

i. Boil the milk and reduce the flame.
ii. Add pre-washed uncooked rice to it and keep cooking till the rice is cooked.
iii. Add sugar to the milk and rice mixture and keep cooking for another 3-4 minutes. Add the nuts, cardamom and saffron leaves to it.

iv. Serve either cold or hot as per your wish.

Calcium content - 300 mg

Indian Fudge with Condensed Milk and Dry Coconut

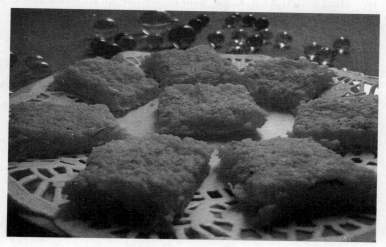

Makes 30 square pieces

Ingredients

Dry desicated coconut	–	250 gm
Sugar	–	250 gm
Milk	–	1500 ml
Ghee	–	2 tbsp
Cardamom powder	–	1½ tbsp
Saffron leaves	–	15 leaves

Method of Preparation

i. Heat the ghee in frying pan on a slow flame.

ii. Add the dry coconut to it. Once warm, take it out and keep it separate.
iii. Boil the milk in a frying pan till it thickens (consistency of churned curd). Add the coconut to it and let it cool in a plate.
iv. Heat a mixture of sugar with about 100 ml of water and cook it for 4-5 minutes. Let it cool.
v. Add the sugar syrup to the coconut mixture.
vi. Put cardamom powder and saffron leaves for flavour.
vii. Put the mixture in a one inch height tray and pat it till it sets.
viii. Once it cools down, cut it into one and half inch squares (about 30 pieces).

Calcium content of one square - 100 mg

Chapter 16
Alternative Therapies

Homeopathy

The word homeopathy is derived from two Greek words 'homoios' meaning similar and 'pathos' meaning disease. It is based on the fact that the substances when taken in crude form produce certain symptoms in the healthy individuals and when given to sick individuals in the potentised form will have a curative effect. It was introduced by a German physician Samuel Hahnemann. It treats the patient as a whole. This system is found effective in treating osteoporosis but it is suggested to consult a qualified homeopath before proceeding for any medication.

Indications of Various Homeopathic Medicines Effective for Osteoporosis

Arnica montana

This is a remedy for the bad effects of mechanical injuries, even if received year's ago. Patient has sore, lame and bruised feeling all through the body. Extremely painful condition that patient can't even bear being touched. It can be taken as long as the pain and the sorenss are present.

Bryonia alba

It is suited to people with rhuematic diathesis.Stitching, tearing pains worse by motion and gets better with rest and lying on painful side.

Calcarea carbonica

It is suited to people with irregular bone development, with curvature of bones especially spine and long bones.It is very effective for diseases arising from defective assimilation and imperfect ossification.Patient feels worse from damp and cold weather.

Calcarea phosphorica

Stiffness, soreness and weakness of the joints affected.It is very well suited for bone spurs.Also effective in case of spinal curvatures especially to the left. It promotes callous formation therefore effective in union of bones.

Eupatorium perfoliatum

It is indicated in case of fever associated with scanty sweat and bony pains. There is bruised sore feeling all over the body as if bones are broken.Pain in neck, head, chest and especially wrists feel as if dislocated.Pains are severe and they come suddenly and go suddenly.

Phosphorus

It is suited to delicate and oversensitive people who gets tired very easily. Patient is very weak and prostrated.Very effective in case of slow healing fractures.There is weakness and burning pain between the shoulder blades.Pains gets worse in cold open air.

Symphytum officinale

It facilitates the union of fractured bones and lessens the peculiar pricking pains. It favours the production of callous. Very effective in cases of mechanical injuries. It relieves the periosteal pain after wounds have healed.

Herbal Medicine

Western herbalism is based on physicians' and herbalists' clinical experience and traditional knowledge of plants with medicinal and curative properties to treat symptoms and diseases and maintain health. For osteoporosis emphasis is on the consumption of calcium containing plants such as horsetail (Equisetum arvense), oat straw (Avena sativa), alfalfa (Medicago sativa), licorice (Glycyrrhiza glabra), marsh mallow (Althaea officinalis), and sourdock (Rumex crispus) etc.

Purple Sage, Red Clover, Liquorice

It aids the working of old joints along with weak digestion, circulatory problems and failing memory. It slows down the ageing process and treats the symptoms accompanying old age.

White Willow

Very effective in case of pain and inflammation. It relieves symptoms that come with gout, arthritis, and stiff joints. Along with other herbs it is a powerful pack for arthritis.

Thyme

It combats the ageing process by maintaining the vitality of the organism. It increases immunity against infections. It helps in relieving bone complaints associated with ageing.

Ginseng

It boosts vitality and releases stress and infection. It makes bones stronger.

Ayurveda

This system of medicine originated in ancient India. In Sanskrit, ayur means life or living, and veda means knowledge, so Ayurveda has been defined as the 'knowledge of living' or the 'science of longevity.' Following are some of the ayurvedic medicines useful for osteoporosis.

Sesame Oil

It helps loosen the stiff joints and thereby pain associated with it. It combats ageing process by improving circulation and rejuvenating the entire body system. It is a rich source of calcium so can be chewed without having any side effects. Pain can also be relieved by massaging sesame oil to the affected parts.

Triphala

Also known as castor oil. It reduces stiffness of joints and bone deformities. Very effective in case of gout. Bone pains improve by application of heat and oil. It relieves low backache associated with anxiety, insomnia and constipation.

Almonds

Almonds soaked overnight in water and blended in the morning with milk proves to be a good source of calcium.

Dandelion Tea

It is very effective in case of osteoporosis as it has the property of increasing bone density. It also aids in reducing weight which in itself is a boon for the affected joints as they will have less weight to bear on them.

Soy

It is very useful for women suffering from osteoporosis. It normalizes the hormonal imbalances the maintains the level of oestrogen so very effective in women suffering from osteoporosis.

Traditional Chinese Medicine (Chinese Herbs)

Chinese herbalism is one of the major components of traditional Chinese medicine (TCM). Chinese herbalism is a holistic medical system ,that is, they treat a patient as a whole both at the mental and spiritual level as well as the physical health of the individual. Illness is seen as a disharmony or imbalance among these aspects of the individual.

Chinese medicine is effective in treating and preventing osteoporosis. According to Chinese medicine practitioners osteoporosis arises due to a decline in kindey Qi or energy. Kidney rules the bones and when there is something wrong with the Kidney, the bones weaken. So, by Chinese medicines we basically treat kidneys.

Postmenopausal osteoporosis is categorized in Chinese medicine as kidney vacuity bone wilting and kidney vacuity lumbar pain. Tai Xi is the foot shao yin kidney channel source point. Shen Shu is the back transport point of the kidneys, while Guan Yuan nourishes and secures the kidneys. Therefore, supplementing these three points has the effect of supplementing the kidneys and boosting the essence. Shen Shu and Guan Yuan is able to increase serum levels of estrogen, thus inhibiting osteoclastosis and promoting osteoblastosis.

Acupuncture at these three points along with calcium and vitamin D supplements increases bone density in postmenopausal women than supplementation of calcium and vitamin D alone. Chinese medicines are effective in promoting faster recovery from traumatic fractures, shortening the period of treatment by as much as one-third to one-half. The natural herbal formulas of traditional Chinese medicine offer promise for treating the root causes of osteoporosis and bone disease, providing the body with a beneficial environment and conditions for maximizing bone health.

Yoga

Yoga is an excellent weight bearing exercise as it stimulates bone building for both the upper and lower body. It ensures that the body receives the required quantity of hormones for maintaining bone strength and health and well being. Regular practice of weight bearing yoga postures build bone strength and avoid this debilitating disease. To build bone mass with yoga and other exercise, it should be practiced at least 30 minutes a day and five days a week.

Simple back bending poses like sphinx, cobra and bridge help to strengthen the spine as well as prevent and correct kyphosis (excessive curvature of the upper spine).It also stimulate the thyroid gland to balance the endocrine system and promotes bone growth.

Start slow with simple yoga poses and gradually build up the length and difficulty of the postures. Gradually increase the intensity of yoga practice.It will help in building stronger bones but it is advised not to push yourself past your edge to reduce any risk of injury.Balancing poses not only build bones but also reduces the risk of falls. Various poses which help preventing osteoporosis are Virasana (Hero Pose), Siddhasana (Adept's Pose), Baddha Konasana (Bound Angle Pose), Janu Sirsasana (Head-to-Knee Forward Bend), Marichyasana III (Pose Dedicated to the Sage Marichi, III), Upavistha Konasana (Wide Angle Pose), and simple squatting.

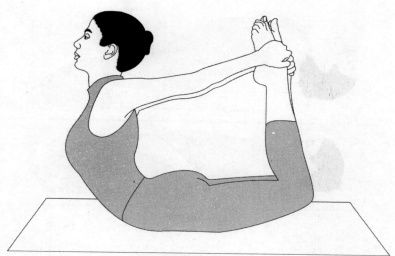
Dhanurasana

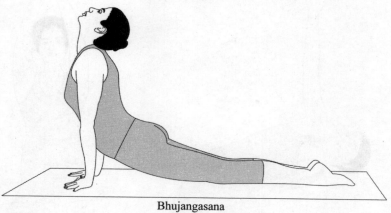
Bhujangasana

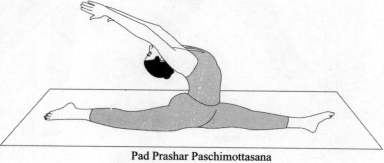
Pad Prashar Paschimottasana

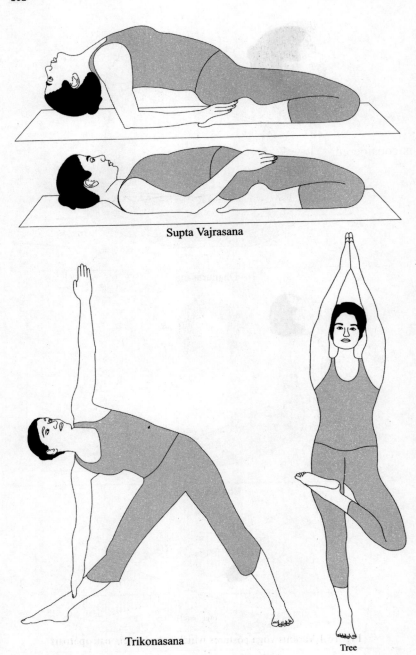

Supta Vajrasana

Trikonasana

Tree

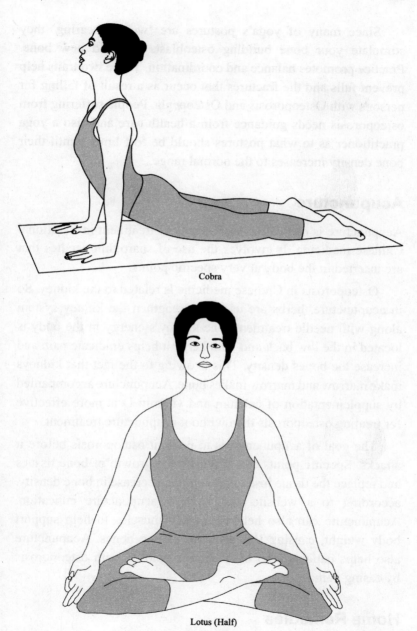

Cobra

Lotus (Half)

Fig. 16.1 Various yoga postures which help prevent osteoporosis

Since many of yoga's postures are 'weight bearing' they stimulate your bone building osteoblasts to build new bone. Practice promotes balance and coordination. These two traits help prevent falls and the fractures that occur as a result of falling for persons with Osteoporosis and Osteopenia. People suffering from osteoporosis needs guidance from a health care and also a yoga practitioner as to what postures should be 'off limits' until their bone density increases to the normal range.

Acupuncture

Acupuncture is one of the main forms of treatment in traditional Chinese medicine. It involves the use of sharp, thin needles that are inserted in the body at very specific points.

Osteoporosis in Chinese medicine is related to the kidney. So in acupuncture, herbs are used to strengthen the kidney system along with needle treatment. The kidney's energy in the body is located in the low back and with herbs it helps eradicate pain and increase the bones density. This is owing to the fact that kidneys make marrow and marrow makes bone. Acupuncture accompanied by supplementation of calcium and vitamin D is more effective for treating osteoporosis than without acupuncture treatment.

The goal of acupuncture is to prevent osteoporosis before it attacks. Specific points can stimulate the growth of bone tissues and replace the tissue loss to prevent the decrease in bone density, according to a website dedicated to acupuncture education. Acupuncture can also help strengthen muscles to help support body weight, causing less pressure on the bones. Acupuncture also helps patients who have been diagnosed with osteoporosis by easing pain.

Home Remedies

To prevent osteoporosis one should drink atleast one cup of milk daily, exercise daily, eat dairy products, avoid caffeine, alcohol and smoking.

Some Home Remedies for Osteoporosis

- **Apples**: Boron is a trace mineral that helps your body hold on to calcium. It even acts as a mild estrogen replacement. Boron is found in apples and other fruits such as pears, grapes, dates, raisins, and peaches. It's also in nuts such as almonds, peanuts, and hazelnuts.
- **Banana**: Eating a banana daily helps to build bones. Studies have found that women who have diets high in potassium also have stronger bones in their spines and hips. It is due to potassium's ability to keep blood healthy and balanced so the body doesn't have to extract calcium from the skeleton to keep blood up to the par.
- **Broccoli**: 1/2 cup broccoli gives daily dose of vitamin K. Very effective in case of postmenopausal women.
- **Orange juice**: Rich source of Vitamin C. It helps in rebuilding bones and preventing osteoporosis.
- **Pineapple juice**: It provides the body with manganese. Manganese deficiency is a predictor of osteoporosis. Other manganese sources are oatmeal, nuts, beans, cereals, spinach, and tea.
- **Salmon and Sardines**: Both of these delicious fishes are high in calcium, and salmon is also a good source of vitamin D.
- **Tofu**: It is a a potential bone strengthener. Soy contains proteins that act like a weak oestrogen in the body. These 'phytoestrogens' or plant based oestrogens, may help women regain bone strength.
- **Yoghurt**: The lactose or sugar in yoghurt, has already been broken down, so people with lactose intolerance can also eat it and get the benefits of the high calcium content.

Appendix 1
National and International Statistics of Osteoporosis

Osteoporosis prevalence

- Affects 200 million women worldwide
  - ½ of women aged 60 to 70
  - ⅔ of women aged 80 or older
- Approximately 30 percent of women over the age of 50 have one or more vertebral fractures
- Approximately one in five men over the age of 50 will have an osteoporosis related fracture in their remaining lifetime

Magnitude of osteoporosis as of today and future predictions

The WHO technical report series 843- assessment of fracture risk and its application to screening for post menopausal osteoporosis predicts significant increase in fracture to neck of femur in Asian population. By 2050 it is likely to be a major demographic factor due to change in lifestyle and increase in survival rate of elderly. The incidence of fracture to neck of femur is likely to increase from 8,40,000 cases in 1986 to 6.26 million cases in 2050 and 71% are likely to occur in developing world. India is likely to have incidence of 1.2 million cases / year. Presently in India, there are about 61 million osteoporotic cases of which 35% are post-menopausal women. Presumably women will bear greater brunt; however problem is also huge in men and likely to increase in future.

Appendix II
Incidence of Osteoporotic Fractures in Women

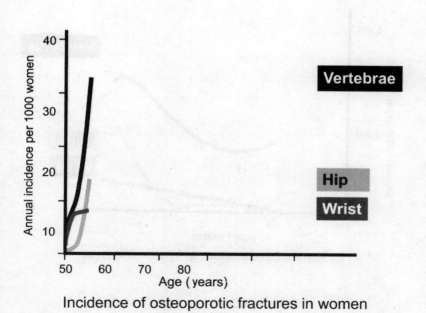

Incidence of osteoporotic fractures in women

Appendix III
Incidence of Osteoporotic Fractures in Men

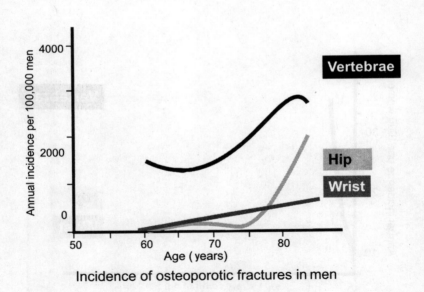

Incidence of osteoporotic fractures in men

Appendix IV
Projected Number of Osteoporotic Hip Fractures Worldwide

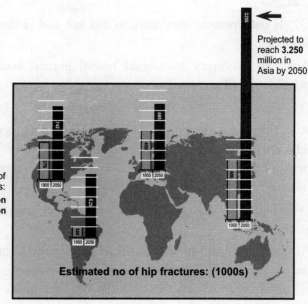

Appendix V
Frequently Asked Questions

Q1. Are vegetarians more prone to osteoporosis?

Ans: No

Q2. Is osteoporosis inevitable in old age and is there no escape from it?

Ans: No. Contrary to normal belief, normal bone density is possible in old age also.

Q3. What is the effect of early menopause on bone health?

Ans: Hormonal changes lead to risk of osteoporosis in all women who are post menopausal, challenge is larger in early menopause because the osteoporosis management has to be done for greater life span.

Q4. Is it a fact that the women who do not bear children have strong bones?

Ans: Yes, it is a fact that during the pregnancy and lactational period the chances for Calcium and Vitamin deficiency are more and that is called Osteomalacia. Along with this Osteoporosis makes the disease commonly called Osteoporomalacia, but bearing children is just one issue and if conscious efforts are done all women can have healthy bones.

Q5. How much milk is required by a body everyday to get adequate Calcium?

Ans: Milk is not the only source of the Calcium in diet. 100 ml of milk gives 200 mg of Calcium. In case of high value milk rich diet 400 to 600 ml of milk is sufficient.

Q6. How many hours do I need to sit in sun for adequate Vitamin D?

Ans: 30 to 40 minutes continuous exposure to sun is considered adequate for normal vitamin D synthesis.

Q7. Should everybody go for BMD checkup?

Ans: No, confirm your risk with IOF risk test.

Q8. If we have fracture do we presume that the orthopaedic surgeon will put us on osteoporosis treatment?

Ans: Unfortunately it doesn't happen always like that, although it is desirable.

Bibliography

i. Reiner Bartl and Bertha Frisch (Osteoporosis; Springer India Pvt Ltd; 2004)
ii. Balusankaran (Osteoporosis; South East Asia Regional Office, WHO; 2000)
iii. M. Swaminathan (Advanced Book on Food and Nutrition Vol 1, 2; Bangalore Printing and Publishing Company Ltd, Bangalore; 2003)
iv. Publication on Exercises 'Move It or Loose it' (International Osteoporosis Foundation; 2005)
v. Bon Apetat (International Osteoporosis Foundation; 2007)
vi. Osteoporosis International (International Osteoporosis Foundation)
vii. Archives of Osteoporosis (International Osteoporosis Foundation)
viii. Progress in Osteoporosis (International Osteoporosis Foundation)
ix. Journal of Bone and Joint Surgery (Am and British Edition)
x. Orthopedic Clinics of North America
xi. Indian Journal of Orthopaedics
xii. Campbell's Operative Orthopaedics 11th Edition
xiii. Chapmans Orthopaedic Surgery 3rd Edition
xiv. Turek's Orthopeadics: Principles and Their Application. 6th Edition
xv. ISBMR publication, Booklet on Nutrition